PRAISE FOR

The
ALLERGY-FREE
Pantry

"With *The Allergy-Free Pantry*, Colette Martin has applied her personal experience and vast knowledge to create a phenomenal resource for preparing and eating safe meals without risking exposure to the top 8 most common food allergens, which is no small task. Readers will not only gain a better understanding of their own food allergies, but will be equipped with new and exciting options for meals and snacks. From preparing your own salad dressing to enjoying allergen-free snickerdoodles, Colette covers all the bases in her wonderful new cookbook!"

—**DAVID STUKUS**, MD, board-certified allergist and
Assistant Professor of Pediatrics at Nationwide Children's Hospital in Columbus, Ohio

"No more fussing over 'may contain' labels; everything from homemade Pancake and Baking Mix to Toaster Tarts with your own Cherry Vanilla Jam is packed into this do-it-yourself dream! *The Allergy-Free Pantry* is a massive resource that reaches every nook and cranny of safe eating, allowing even beginner cooks to step into their kitchen with confidence."

—**ALISA FLEMING**, Founder of GoDairyFree.org, Senior Editor of *Allergic Living* Magazine

"Colette Martin knows that when you're feeding a family with multiple food allergies, the best—and safest—way to enjoy the foods you love is to make them from scratch at home. From toaster tarts to shepherd's pie to brownie bites, *The Allergy-Free Pantry* serves up kid-friendly recipes that cover breakfast, snacks, main meals, and desserts. But you'll especially appreciate Martin's guidance on substitutions for common allergens such as dairy and eggs, as well as how to make allergen-free versions of pantry staples that can form the foundation of your family's cooking, whether from the pages of this book or another beloved recipe."

—**KELLI AND PETER BRONSKI**, coauthors of *Gluten-Free Family Favorites* and
Artisanal Gluten-Free Cooking

"*The Allergy-Free Pantry* takes the guesswork out of cooking for a restricted diet, and opens up new doors for novice chefs and old pros alike! Packed with easy-to-follow recipes, including those that are hard to come by in the world of allergy-free fare (hamburger buns, croutons, toaster tarts, and so much more!), this cookbook is a must-have for anyone avoiding common food allergens."

—**MARY JO STROBEL**, Executive Director, American Partnership for Eosinophilic Disorders

THE EXPERIMENT

BECAUSE EVERY BOOK IS A TEST OF NEW IDEAS

"*The Allergy-Free Pantry* is a must-have for anyone living with food allergies. Colette Martin demystifies the often-confounding world of 'substitutions,' enabling home cooks to take back control over the ingredients in their food. In the pages of this book, you will find many ingenious ways to mix up everything you need for a well-stocked pantry, plus a wealth of new recipes that use your new tool kit. Whether you want to can it, jam it, blend it, dress it, sauce it, bake it, or cook it, there's something in here for you."

—CYBELE PASCAL, author of *Allergy-Free and Easy Cooking* and *The Allergen-Free Baker's Handbook* and founder of Cybele's Free-to-Eat

"Anyone with multiple food reactions should buy this book! I can't tell you how many patients I see whose lives Colette Martin has changed. *The Allergy-Free Pantry* is an excellent resource."

—DR. STEPHEN WANGEN, Medical Director, IBS Treatment Center

"Colette Martin is a dedicated food allergy mother and advocate who has spent over a decade developing recipes for delicious allergen-free meals. By sharing her insight and creations with us in *The Allergy-Free Pantry*, Colette once again helps us greatly expand the breadth of options we can serve our food-allergic children. Thanks to Colette, we don't have to compromise on taste or nutrition."

—PAUL ANTICO, founder and CEO of AllergyEats, food allergy advocate, and father of three food-allergic children

"A diagnosis of food allergy means that many favorite meals, snacks, and condiments become off-limits. *The Allergy-Free Pantry* is a guide book for you to learn how to replace those favorites with safe, made-at-home versions of foods you thought you'd have to give up. Colette's how-to style will give even a novice cook or baker a way to become confident in the kitchen."

—LYNDA MITCHELL, Vice President, Kids With Food Allergies, a division of the Asthma and Allergy Foundation of America

"I am humbled by Colette Martin's commitment and applaud her hard work, her spirit, and the contents of this book. As a chef and advocate, I look forward to implementing some of the recipes from *The Allergy-Free Pantry* here in the South Point kitchens."

—KEITH NORMAN, Assistant Executive Chef and Food Safety Manager at South Point Hotel, Casino, and Spa

"For anyone who has asked, 'What do I do now?' after a child is diagnosed with multiple life-threatening food allergies, Colette Martin has the answer. She provides a guide to the alternate universe of feeding a food-allergy family in steps so logical that they would make anyone a better cook. Follow Colette and your family won't miss a thing in flavor, variety, and nutrition."

—HENRY EHRLICH, editor of asthmaallergieschildren.com and author of *Food Allergies: Traditional Chinese Medicine, Western Science, and the Search for a Cure*

"Finally! Thanks to Colette Martin, the food allergy community can make all of our culinary cravings and necessities, from meals to savory snacks to baking staples. With precise explanations, the recipes in *The Allergy-Free Pantry* are easily approachable. And no, Colette Martin doesn't build concepts around short-lived, pre-processed 'substitute' foods. Her back-to-the-basics cooking approach offers those of us contending with multiple food allergies and restrictions the means to eat like the rest of the world . . . and possibly even better."

—SUSAN WEISSMAN, author of *Feeding Eden*

COLETTE MARTIN

The ALLERGY-FREE Pantry

MAKE YOUR OWN STAPLES, SNACKS, AND MORE
WITHOUT WHEAT, GLUTEN, DAIRY,
EGGS, SOY OR NUTS

THE EXPERIMENT
NEW YORK

THE ALLERGY-FREE PANTRY: *Make Your Own Staples, Snacks, and More without Wheat, Gluten, Dairy, Eggs, Soy or Nuts*

The Experiment, LLC
220 East 23rd Street, Suite 301
New York, NY 10010-4674
www.theexperimentpublishing.com

This book is not intended to provide medical
advice. While care was taken to provide correct
and helpful information, the suggestions in this
book are not intended as dietary advice or as a
substitute for consulting a dietician, physician,
or other medical professional. It is the reader's
sole responsibility to determine which foods
are appropriate and safe for his or her family
to consume. The author and publisher make no
claims regarding the presence of food allergens
and disclaim all liability in connection with the
use of this book.

The Experiment's books are available at special
discounts when purchased in bulk for premiums
and sales promotions as well as for fund-raising
or educational use. For details, contact us at info@
theexperimentpublishing.com.

Library of Congress Cataloging-in-Publication Data

Martin, Colette (Colette F.)
   The allergy-free pantry : make your own staples,
snacks, and more without wheat, gluten, dairy, eggs, soy
or nuts / Colette Martin.
      pages cm
   Includes index.
   ISBN 978-1-61519-208-3 (pbk.) -- ISBN 978-1-61519-209-0
(ebook) 1. Food allergy--Diet therapy--Recipes. I. Title.
   RC588.D53M368 2014
   641.5'6318--dc23
                                  2014010752

ISBN 978-1-61519-208-3
Ebook ISBN 978-1-61519-209-0

Cover design by Joanna Williams
Cover photographs by Colette Martin
Author photograph by Harry Yudenfriend
Text design by Pauline Neuwirth, Neuwirth &
Associates, Inc.

Manufactured in the United States of America
Distributed by Workman Publishing Company, Inc.
Distributed simultaneously in Canada by Thomas Allen
& Son Ltd.

First printing August 2014
10 9 8 7 6 5 4 3 2 1

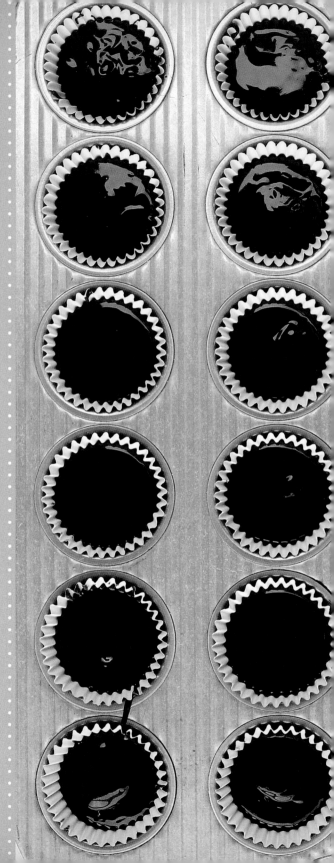

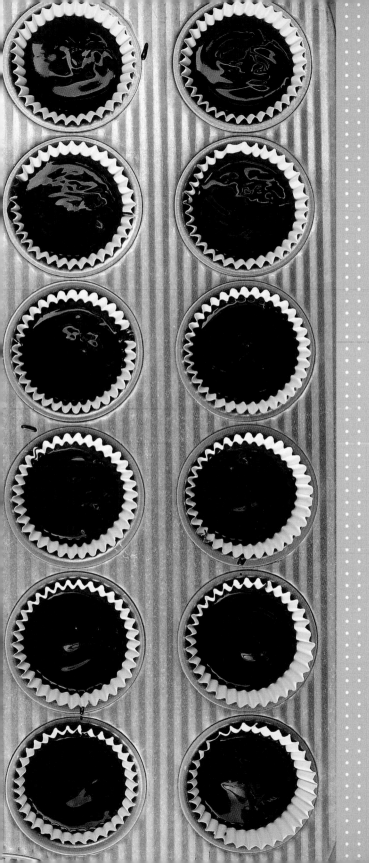

For Kevin,
The sun shines
wherever you are.

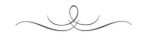

CONTENTS

INTRODUCTION

When you or someone in your family has food allergies your first challenge after diagnosis is to find safe, healthy foods to fill your pantry. You want to be able to make the foods you crave. You long to be free of processed foods and the stress of constantly reading labels. You need extreme control over the ingredients in your food.

I know how hard it is to find foods for a family with multiple food allergies. When my son was diagnosed with allergies to wheat, dairy, eggs, soy, and peanuts, I had to throw out most of the food in my pantry and start over. For years I searched the shelves at the grocery store for the one package of cookies that just might be safe for my son. Then, still uncertain, I would call the manufacturer and ask questions; sometimes I found a satisfactory answer and sometimes I didn't. I religiously stuck to the few brands I had determined were safe and celebrated every new product those companies introduced.

Luckily, it's easier to find allergen-free and gluten-free products today. The CDC estimates that food allergies in children have risen 50 percent between 1999 and 2011.[*] The silver lining in this extreme rise in food allergies is that both small and large food vendors are scrambling to meet the needs of our community. I am grateful for them. Yet while these foods have helped my family cope, they are often laden with empty calories and preservatives. For many with food allergies, they still contain forbidden ingredients, and they can be expensive and hard to find.

An increasing number of families are dealing with what I call "extreme" food allergies; instead of five foods to avoid, some have a family member with only a dozen foods they *can* eat. Some families have a short list of foods to avoid, but the list includes less common allergens. If rice is on your list, nearly every off-the-shelf solution is not an option for you. When corn is on your list, reading labels gets ten times harder.[†] And a growing number of us are becoming more conscious of the amount of sugar and high carbohydrate counts, genetically modified ingredients (GMOs), and preservatives in our food. Some with food allergies must avoid all preservatives and food coloring, yet additives such as FD&C Blue #1 or FD&C Red #3 (and other numbered "foods") are considered safe by the US federal agency that regulates our food.

---

[*] NCHS Data Brief No. 121, May 2013, http://www.cdc.gov/nchs/data/databriefs/db121.pdf.

[†] The Food Allergen Labeling and Consumer Protection Act of 2004 requires that only the top eight food allergens (wheat, dairy, eggs, soy, peanuts, tree nuts, fish, and shellfish) be clearly labeled, using the common name.

Mealtime, snack time, and any occasion involving food can be very stressful for those dealing with food allergies. Whether you need to avoid one food or dozens of foods, you will find solutions in this book. Your relationship with food will become much easier when you take back control over the ingredients in your food.

I must confess that I fed my children store-bought chocolate doughnuts and peanut butter and jelly sandwiches until food allergies disrupted our lives. My family missed those foods and I know yours does too. Many of you have told me that you wish your kids could experience a Pop-Tart, that your children have never tasted a Tootsie Roll, or that you just need one really great egg-free mayonnaise that you can rely on. The good news is you *can* have allergen-free versions of these items, and I will show you how to make them—in the safety of your own kitchen.

It can be scary to make new recipes for the first time, but you will be pleasantly surprised to discover how easy it is to make healthy, safe pantry staples at home. Whether you are a novice in the kitchen or simply need new techniques and ingredients, you will find the guidance you need in this book. If *The Allergy-Free Pantry* is your first food-allergy cookbook, you're in the right place! The pantry staples you'll learn to make here can be used (in lieu of the store-bought versions) with the recipes in other cookbooks. If you already have a food-allergy cookbook, such as *Learning to Bake Allergen-Free*, the techniques you learned there will apply to the recipes in this book.

The most important component of healthy eating for those with food allergies—a category in which I include those who are at risk for anaphylaxis,* suffer from celiac disease or other autoimmune conditions, or are intolerant to certain foods—is to avoid the foods that make you sick. I know that many of you have allergies beyond gluten, wheat, dairy, eggs, soy, and nuts; to help you with that I have made the recipes as flexible as possible. I give you permission to substitute where it makes sense, and I insist that you do so when needed to avoid an allergen.

This book starts with the staples that everyone needs in their pantry (a word I use throughout this text to include cupboards, shelves, the refrigerator, and the freezer—anywhere you might store the ingredients you need to cook and bake). Instead of picking up milk, eggs, and bread at the convenience store, I will teach you how to make your own non-dairy milk and what to use in place of eggs (and when to use them), and I will share the secrets to wheat-free and gluten-free flour blends so that you can make the perfect Sandwich Bread (page 51).

Next, you will find recipes to replace processed foods. If you need an alternative to traditional peanut butter, I'll give you a lesson on how to make your own Sunflower Seed Butter (page 77). I will show you how to make jam without pectin or preservatives, with an amount of sugar you control. I won't force you to learn how to preserve jams—you have the option to make them to eat now and in the next week or two—but if you want to learn, I'll show you how.

---

* Anaphylaxis is a rapidly progressing, life-threatening allergic reaction to an antigen (in the case of food allergies, usually a protein).

It is surprisingly simple to make salad dressing. Instead of teaching you how to read the labels of 209 bottles of salad dressing (yes, I counted) on the shelf at the grocery store, I will teach you to shake up your own in minutes. Some recipes took a lot of experimenting and creativity; my quest for a dairy-free, soy-free, egg-free mayonnaise caused me to waste a great deal of oil and lose a lot of sleep trying to invent a method, but the journey was worth it. Now that I make my own "mayonnaise," I will never go back to the one ultra-expensive allergen-free version I can only sometimes find on the shelf.

What's on the menu for breakfast, lunch, and dinner? In Part 2 (page 115) you will find the recipes you need to reduce mealtime stress. Options for breakfast include cereals, English Muffins (page 131), and yes, even those coveted Toaster Tarts (page 129). There are side dishes that will take you from the dinner table to the picnic blanket. Whether you crave French Fries (page 159) or Onion Rings (page 163), you are covered and there is no need to worry about what was made in the same fryer. I encourage you to experiment with different toppings on the Perfect Pizza Crust (page 181), and I'll even show you how to make your own pasta. The meals in this book are designed so that you can make some for now and save some (or freeze some) for later.

And let's not forget snacks. Instead of opening an expensive package of chocolate chip cookies that might go stale within a few days, I'll show you how to make cookie dough rolls for about two-thirds the cost,* and you will be able to slice and bake just as many cookies as you need, when you need them. If your wheat-allergic son is craving pretzels or your nut-allergic daughter needs a treat for school on short notice, you will find both savory and sweet treats in Part 3 (page 201) that fit the bill.

As I developed these recipes I was conscious of the fact that you don't have a lot of spare time. If I couldn't make it easily, or if the store-bought version was healthy, affordable, and easy to find, I didn't include it. Some of these recipes require elapsed time but little hands-on time; others require a bit more of your attention.

You may be wondering if a home-crafted jam in a Ball jar is as worthy as a jar of Smucker's, or whether a homemade cookie is inferior to the Oreo or the treat bought at Starbucks. I too have been suspicious of homemade food in jars. It might take some adjustment to get used to the idea that the crackers you made and stashed in your pantry are just as good—and quite possibly better than—the version you might buy at the store. You *can* take back control over the ingredients that go into your food, and you will have the peace of mind of knowing that you made it yourself with trusted ingredients.

As you embark on this mission to create an allergy-free pantry in your own home, you will find that instead of just one safe option for the member of your family with food allergies, your cupboard, refrigerator, and freezer will soon be full of delicious, healthy foods the whole family will enjoy. Embrace the journey!

---

* Cost will vary depending on the ingredients and brands that are safe for you to use.

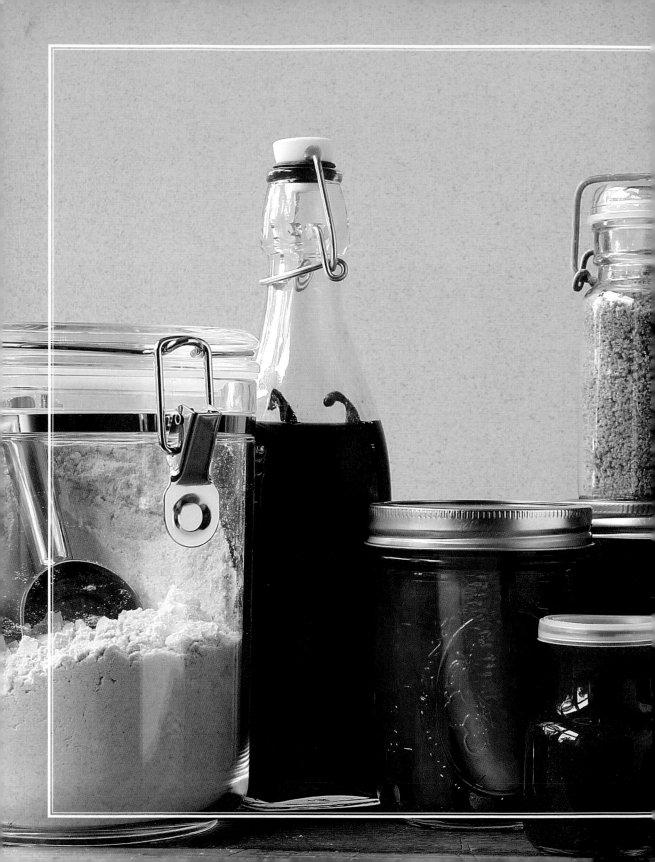

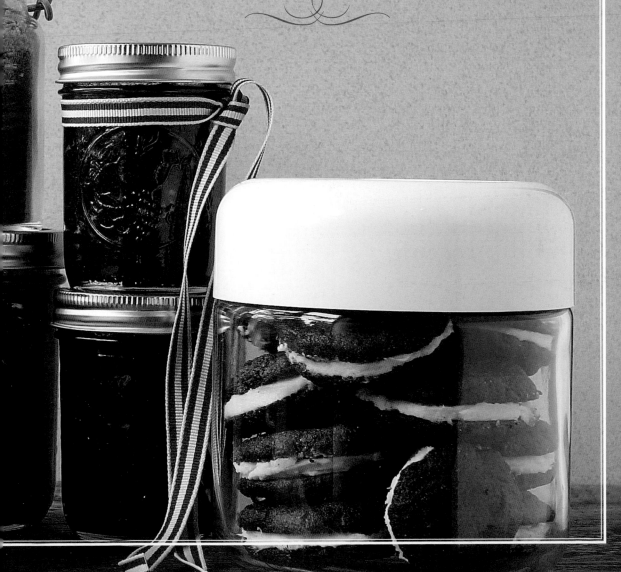

PART 1

ESSENTIALS

1.

Getting Started

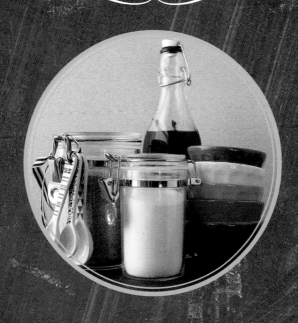

You are on a journey to create a safe pantry and avoid the foods you or your family are allergic to. Whether that includes just one food or dozens, the journey starts by stocking the pantry with basic items that will be used on a weekly—if not daily—basis. To do so, you must first understand how to find safe ingredients.

I am encouraging you to make food at home, but I am not asking you to let your guard down when it comes to safety. You still need to ensure that the ingredients you buy are safe for you and your family. If a product has a label, you must scrutinize it. You must avoid open bins, scrub the produce you bring home, and be very careful with homemade foods made by well-meaning friends and family—only accept those that you have vetted and are certain will be safe. You must always choose only ingredients that avoid all of your family's food allergens, following your doctor's instructions.

In this chapter you will learn about the ingredients and tools to use, with tips on how to choose the best options for you and your family.

AVOIDING CONTAMINATION

While you won't be buying a lot of processed foods (instead, you will be making food at home), there are some staples that you need to purchase and there may be times when you choose to buy an item off the shelf. To find safe products—products that do not contain the foods you or your family are allergic to—you must read the ingredients labels.

The Food Allergen Labeling and Consumer Protection Act of 2004 (FALCPA) in the United States requires that the ingredients label on all packaged foods must clearly state, using the common terms, any of the top eight food allergens that the food contains. For example, if a product contains milk (dairy) or a component of milk (e.g., *whey* or *casein*), the ingredient must be listed as *milk* (and not simply *whey* or

casein) either in the detailed ingredients list or in a "contains" statement directly below the detailed ingredients. Products may also contain advisory labels (e.g., "may contain nuts" or "processed in a facility that also processes soy"), but these warnings are optional and the language is not standardized; this means that you must always read the detailed ingredients.

If the list of foods you need to avoid goes beyond the top eight food allergens—wheat, milk, eggs, soy, peanuts, tree nuts, fish, and shellfish—reading ingredients labels is much harder. Ingredients such as *hydrolyzed vegetable protein* or *natural flavor* need to be investigated further to determine what they really are. You must work with your doctor to understand your complete list of foods to avoid.

In addition to the ingredients that are intended to be in the food you buy (i.e., what is listed on the ingredients label), processed foods can sometimes become contaminated when they are made in the same facility or on shared equipment with ingredients you are allergic to. Again, the advisory labels for this possibility are optional. The best way to find out what is processed on shared equipment or in the same facility is to call the manufacturer and ask. Be sure to always choose only foods that are safe for you and your family. If you aren't sure (or don't get a satisfactory answer), leave the product on the shelf.

In 2013, the FDA issued guidance on the use of the term *gluten-free* on product labels.[*] Starting in late 2014, food manufacturers

---

* U.S. Food and Drug Administration. "Gluten-Free Labeling of Foods." Last modified November 6, 2013. http://www.fda.gov/food/guidanceregulation/guidancedocumentsregulatoryinformation/allergens/ucm362510.htm

may use the wording *gluten-free* on a product label only if the product is inherently gluten-free, does not contain a gluten grain (wheat, barley, or rye), or contains less than 20 parts per million (ppm) of gluten. This labeling is optional, and (unlike the labeling requirements for food allergens) there is no requirement to state whether a product *does* contain gluten. Those who must avoid gluten must still read detailed ingredients labels and investigate suspicious ingredients.

Contamination (sometimes referred to as cross-contamination or cross-contact) can also occur at the grocery store. Always purchase packaged items rather than those in open bins. It's too easy for the scoop from the nut bin to be left in the seed bin, or the spoon from the olives at the salad bar to be dipped into the cheese. Spices, seeds, and cereals also fall into this category.

Once you have brought safe food home from the market you need to make sure it stays safe and avoid contamination within your home. If you can't completely eliminate food allergens from your home, you must take precautions. Sponges, kitchen towels, utensils, and appliances are just a few of the places where contamination can occur. You may decide to designate certain zones as safe. For example, don't use the same sponge to clean your food-allergic son's high chair tray that you used to wipe up wheat bread crumbs. Don't use the same blender to make hemp milk as you did to make a smoothie using cow's milk. You may need to set aside certain appliances, pans, and baking dishes for safe cooking, and keep them stored in a separate location. Avoid utensils, tools, and cutting boards made from wood or other porous materials. I recommend paper towels and frequent use of the dishwasher. Always take precautions to stay safe.

INGREDIENTS AND SUBSTITUTIONS

One size doesn't fit all when it comes to food allergies. My son is allergic to wheat, milk, eggs, soy, and peanuts. I am allergic to soy and gluten. While my son and I are allergic to soy, we are both able to tolerate soy fats (soybean oil and soy lecithin). Food allergies are most often due to the protein in food, but your doctor may advise you to avoid the fats as well.

You will have your own list of foods to avoid. If you are doing an elimination diet to determine which foods to avoid or doing trials to add foods back into your diet, you may need to make a recipe with one set of ingredients this week and a different set of ingredients next week.

You must always follow your doctor's advice, but you don't always need to follow my recipes to the letter. I have developed them to be as flexible as possible. For some ingredients (e.g., oils and non-dairy milks) I have chosen what I prefer, but these are easily replaced with other options. For other ingredients (e.g., shortening) you have the option to choose what works best for you. Here and in the next few chapters, I will explain the ingredients and note some substitutions that you may need to make.

While some brand names are mentioned throughout this text, always check the detailed ingredients label every time you use a product; ingredients *do* change.

CHOOSING SHORTENING AND OILS

Nearly every baked recipe will call for some type of fat—either shortening or oil. While the proteins in food trigger most food allergies, an increasing number of people are being advised to avoid oils derived from the foods to which they are allergic. You must select the products that are safe for you, following your doctor's advice.

Shortening can replace the butter used in traditional recipes; the best-performing shortening products remain solid at room temperature. When a recipe calls for chilled or cold shortening, use it straight from the refrigerator (except for palm fruit oil, as noted below). If a recipe calls for softened shortening, let it sit at room temperature for at least 2 hours before using it. You may choose from a variety of options:

Earth Balance Natural Shortening—This is one of my favorite shortenings (with a combination of palm fruit, canola, soybean, flax, and olive oils—all non-GMO) due to its superior performance. If your doctor has advised you to avoid any of these ingredients, choose another option.

Coconut oil—Coconut oil can be used whenever a recipe calls for shortening (as long as you are not allergic to it). There are many brands of coconut oil; look for one that is highly refined and cold-pressed to avoid a strong coconut taste.

Palm fruit oil—Spectrum Organic All Vegetable Shortening is an example of palm fruit oil that works well in baking and for making frosting. Always use it at room temperature even if the recipe calls for chilled or cold shortening, as it will stiffen too much to work with after refrigerating. Note that this ingredient is not identical to palm oil.

If you are not allergic to milk, you may substitute butter, in equal amounts, whenever a recipe calls for shortening.

If none of these options work for you, you may need to turn to one of the softer "spreads" to use when the recipe calls for shortening. I don't recommend choosing a spread when making frostings or syrups (if you have no other safe options go ahead, but recognize that the results may not be ideal), but they can be used (well chilled) to make cookies and pie crusts. If you are substituting a spread for softened shortening, allow it to sit at room temperature for just 30 minutes. Some options include:

Earth Balance Organic Coconut Spread—This product contains coconut and palm fruit oils, as well as sunflower lecithin and other ingredients.

Earth Balance Soy Free Buttery Spread—This combination of palm fruit, canola, safflower, and olive oils contains no soy proteins or fats.

Homemade Buttery Spread—If you're up for making your own spread (or need to), the Homemade Buttery Spread recipe (page 37) allows you to combine flaxseed meal and coconut oil with other oils of your choice.

You have a lot of flexibility to substitute (in equal amounts) when a recipe calls for oil.

Also, if a recipe calls for melted shortening you may substitute oil.

Oils—Oils are usually single-ingredient products, making it easier to select a safe option. In recipes I specify my preferred oil for that item, but any oil may be substituted in equal amounts. Options include sunflower, grapeseed, safflower, and canola. Light olive oil is a great choice for some breads, pasta, and salad dressings. Changing the type of oil used may affect the taste. Choose organic oil if you wish to ensure that it does not contain genetically modified ingredients.

THE SCOOP ON SUGAR

Sugar is a sweet but tricky subject. I have been asked why my recipes for baked goods don't have options to be made sugar-free. The simple answer is that I am substituting so many other things—gluten-free flours for wheat flour, shortening for butter, flaxseeds and fruit purees for eggs—and sugar is the one ingredient from traditional baking that most of us can still use. There are many medical conditions that require avoiding sugar, but food allergy is rarely one of them. Instead of reducing calories, most with food allergies need to add calories to their diet.

Nevertheless, too many recipes call for excessive amounts of sugar. My approach is to use sugar in moderation and to choose natural and less-processed versions of sugar where possible. The steering wheel is in your hands when it comes to sugar; if you want to add sugar to your Hemp Milk (page 31), it's up to you!

Here are the types of crystal sugar we'll be working with:

Maple sugar—This natural sugar is the crystallized form of maple syrup.

Organic cane sugar—This is usually my first choice when a recipe calls for sugar because it hasn't been chemically processed, bleached, or sprayed with pesticides. You may substitute traditional cane sugar whenever a recipe calls for organic cane sugar, in equal amounts.

Organic light brown sugar—This crystal form of sugar has had some of the molasses (removed during processing) added back in. Traditional light brown sugar may be substituted.

Sucanat—This is whole cane sugar that retains all of its natural molasses. Sucanat may be substituted for either organic cane sugar or brown sugar, in equal amounts.

Turbinado (also known as raw cane sugar)—This is used for creating sugary toppings on cookies or pie crusts.

Liquid sugars are used in some recipes. These can be substituted for crystal forms of sugar (e.g., organic cane sugar) if preferred (with the exception of brown rice syrup and except when creaming). Keep in mind that sugar liquefies when heated. If you choose a liquid sugar over a crystal form of sugar, substitute in equal amounts and do not change the ratio of liquid to dry ingredients; you may need to increase the baking time by a few minutes.

Agave nectar—Agave nectar is a processed sweetener that comes from the cactus-like agave plant. It can be substituted for honey.

Brown rice syrup—This sweetener is derived from culturing cooked rice to break down the starches; the result is a thick sugary substance used as a thickener. It is about half as sweet as sugar. I don't recommend substituting it for other sugars in recipes. Corn syrup (not high-fructose corn syrup) or other sugar syrups may be substituted for brown rice syrup.

Honey—Honey comes in many flavors (depending on which flowers the bees have visited), and locally sourced versions of honey can be quite nice to have in your pantry.

Maple syrup—This natural option can often be locally sourced and is best used in baked goods that benefit from maple's intense flavor. Always choose pure maple syrup over pancake syrup—most pancake syrups have very little maple syrup in them and are loaded with processed sugar and preservatives.

OTHER INGREDIENTS

Baking powder—Gluten-free and egg-free baking requires the use of more baking powder than traditional baking, to assist with leavening. Baking powder usually contains a starch—most often corn starch—but some are formulated with wheat or potato starch. If you must avoid wheat or gluten, be sure to choose baking powder that is wheat-free or gluten-free. If you must avoid corn, Hain Pure Foods Featherweight Baking Powder is made with potato starch. Always choose double-acting baking powder.

Baking soda—Baking soda is a single ingredient—calcium carbonate—and is used in recipes that contain an acid or that don't require the double-acting powers of baking powder.

Cereals—Erewhon organic cereals are a great choice when a recipe calls for gluten-free crisped rice cereal or corn flakes. Choose unsweetened cereal.

Cheese substitutes—Where I use a cheese substitute in a recipe, it is optional. If you would like a product that melts (as cheese does) to top your pasta or pizza, the Daiya brand alternatives are the best I have found.

Chia seeds—Chia seeds are used in whole form. They may be used in place of flaxseed meal, if needed.

Chocolate chips—Chocolate is naturally dairy-free and nut-free, yet chocolate is often processed in the same facility as milk or nuts. Some dairy-free and nut-free chocolate chips contain soy lecithin (if you are allergic to soy, check with your doctor to determine whether you must avoid soy lecithin). One company that makes chocolate chips in a variety of sizes that are completely nut-free, dairy-free, and soy-free is Enjoy Life.

Cocoa—When a recipe calls for cocoa, choose natural unsweetened cocoa powder (rather than Dutch processed); make sure it is labeled 100 percent cocoa (or 100 percent cacao).

Flaxseeds and flaxseed meal—I prefer golden flaxseeds to brown flaxseeds as they don't leave specks of color in the food, but they are interchangeable. You may grind whole flaxseeds into flaxseed meal, or choose pre-ground flaxseed meal.

Hemp seeds—Choose unshelled hemp seeds (sometimes called hemp hearts). Whereas some may mistakenly believe that hemp is marijuana (due to the Controlled Substances Act of 1970 that lumped the two crops together), they are different. Hemp contains no psychoactive ingredients.

Oatmeal—Choose old-fashioned oats and make sure they are certified gluten-free if you are allergic to wheat.

Powdered rice milk—I suggest Better Than Milk Vegan Rice Powder because it is dairy-free, but check the label to make sure it's safe for you. Substitute for this ingredient carefully if you have a milk allergy, as many powdered milks (including powdered coconut milk) contain dairy.

Salt—Salt is used in recipes for taste and also acts as a preservative. Always choose kosher salt or sea salt instead of iodized table salt; the iodine affects the taste.

Sunflower seeds—Choose shelled, unsalted seeds. Raw seeds are best for making Sunflower Milk (page 31), whereas roasted seeds should be used for Sunflower Seed Butter (page 77).

Vanilla beans and vanilla extract—If you choose to make Vanilla Extract (page 288) you will need high-quality vanilla beans. Choose premium, whole vanilla beans. Larger packages will reduce the cost. Store them in the pantry in an airtight container for up to a year. Off-the-shelf vanilla extract may be substituted; be sure to choose one that is gluten-free if you are allergic to wheat.

Vegetables, fruits, and herbs—Always choose fresh, ripe fruit and vegetables and wash them well. When possible, use fresh herbs, but dried herbs may be substituted. When a recipe calls for dried fruit, choose unsweetened. Always check the ingredients labels for dried fruit, dried herbs, and spices to make sure they are safe for you.

Vinegars and acids—Salad dressings, jams, and some baked goods recipes call for an acid. Apple cider vinegar, brown rice vinegar, lemon juice, and plain white vinegar can be substituted for each other in baked goods (in equal amounts). Always wash lemon skins before zesting or juicing to remove oils or wax that may have been used on the skins. If you need to substitute for lemon juice in jams, choose lime juice, orange juice, or apple cider vinegar. Save balsamic vinegar and wine vinegar for salad dressings; substitute brown rice vinegar if you must avoid grapes or sulfites.

Yeast—My recipes that call for yeast specify quick-rising yeast (also known as rapid-rise or fast-acting yeast). In gluten-free baking there is no need for the longer rise times that active dry yeast requires. Yeast will last for a year or longer in the freezer and up to six months in the refrigerator. Bring it to room temperature before using.

EQUIPMENT

Throughout this book you will find tool tips to help you with the recipes. In addition, you will want to keep these items near your allergy-free pantry:

Airtight containers—Ingredients and finished baked goods will be stored in airtight containers. Choose freezer-safe and dishwasher-safe containers made from nonporous materials. Zip-top plastic bags may also be used.

Baking dishes and pans—You will need assorted baking dishes and pans, including a 24-cup mini-muffin pan, a 12-cup standard muffin pan, a 9-inch (23 cm) square baking dish, a 7 by 9-inch (18 by 23 cm) baking dish, a 9 by 12-inch (23 by 30 cm) baking dish, a large 13 by 18-inch (33 by 46 cm) baking sheet (some recipes require two baking sheets or they can be made in two batches), a 13-inch (33 cm) round pizza pan, a gluten-free bread pan that measures 9 by 4 by 4-inches (23 by 10 by 10 cm), and a standard 9 by 5-inch (23 by 13 cm) loaf pan.

Blender—A high-speed blender or food processor is required for making milk and grinding flour and is beneficial in many other recipes.

Cooling rack—It's important to remove baked goods from their vessels promptly after taking them out of the oven, to avoid moisture buildup.

Electric mixer—Recipes that specify high-speed mixing require either a stand mixer or a handheld electric mixer. The stand mixer has the benefit of allowing you to do other prep work while you are mixing. Unless otherwise specified, the paddle blade should be used; dough hooks are not designed for use with gluten-free grains.

Glass canning jars—Assorted canning jars will be needed if you choose to preserve foods using a water bath. I recommend 8- and 4-ounce (240 and 120 ml) jars for jam and 16-ounce (480 ml) jars for pickles and sauces. I suggest buying extra canning lids as well as plastic lids for covering after the jars have been opened. These jars are also ideal for storing bread crumbs, seed butters, syrups, and more.

Immersion blender—A simple, single-speed immersion blender, along with a working glass or the container that comes with the blender, is required to create the perfect mayonnaise and other emulsions. It has the right amount of power and it's easy to trickle in the oils as you blend.

Measuring cups and spoons—Both wet (preferably heat-resistant glass) and dry measuring cups are needed, along with standard-sized measuring spoons.

Mixing bowls and prep bowls—These include small- and medium-sized prep bowls or ramekins as well as mixing bowls of various sizes, including at least one large (4-quart/3.8 liters or larger) bowl for mixing flour blends.

Working glasses (designed to be used with immersion blenders) are ideally suited to some recipes. I also recommend a large stainless-steel bowl for preparing dough.

Non-reactive pan—You will need a medium non-reactive pan to boil jam, fruit butters, and sauces. Aluminum and copper react with acids and should be avoided. Tri-ply stainless steel is my preference.

Other pans—A variety of stovetop pans will be used, including small and medium saucepans, a medium pan with high sides for frying, a medium skillet, a large skillet, and a large pot or Dutch oven.

Parchment paper—Parchment paper serves a dual purpose: it provides a nonstick surface, and it helps to avoid contamination. I prefer pre-cut half sheets of parchment to fit a large (13 by 18-inch/33 by 46 cm) baking sheet.

Spray bottle or oil mister—The simplest way to grease a pan is with a few drops of oil from a spray mister. Alternatively, you may grease a pan or baking dish with a few drops of oil on a paper towel. Note that commercial nonstick cooking sprays usually contain soy lecithin (as always, be sure to check with your doctor to see if it is safe for you). Fill the mister with an oil that is safe for you.

Toaster oven—I suggest the use of a toaster oven for toasting allergen-free bread and reheating allergen-free baked goods that have been frozen. I don't recommend reheating these baked goods in the microwave, as they will take on a spongy quality. If you choose to use a pop-up toaster, designate a separate toaster for allergen-free toasting (to avoid contamination).

Whisks—A 5- to 7-inch (13 to 18 cm) whisk with a small head will be needed to create flaxseed eggs and to mix commercial egg replacers. A standard-sized whisk will be needed to mix batters and salad dressings.

Many of these tools have small crevices where food particles can hide. The best way to avoid contamination is to designate specific tools for allergen-free use only. Steer clear of tools and surfaces made of porous materials, such as wooden rolling pins and cutting boards; choose easy-to-clean materials such as melamine, glass, and stainless steel.

STORAGE CONSIDERATIONS

Throughout the recipes in this book you will find suggestions for storing, refrigerating, freezing, and preserving food, where applicable. Nevertheless, there are some basic rules that apply across the board.

Baked items are always best fresh. After completely cooling, store them in dry, airtight containers in the pantry. Baked goods that won't be eaten within a few days should be frozen and later thawed and/or reheated when it's time to eat them.

Gluten-free bread tends to pick up moisture. Store bread and rolls in airtight containers or plastic bags at room temperature for up to 3 days or in the refrigerator for up to a week. Bread and rolls that will not be eaten within a few days will be best toasted or reheated prior to eating. Bread can also be stored in the freezer for months. I recommend slicing bread prior to freezing and then taking out portions as you need them. Once frozen, bread will be best toasted. Likewise, frozen rolls will be best reheated.

Preserved foods, including jams, ketchup, and pickles, will be shelf-stable for up to a year.

Most homemade milk from seeds and grains will last longer than dairy milk in the refrigerator—up to 3 weeks—but are best when used within a week. Always shake them well before using.

Gluten-free flours, once opened, are best stored in airtight containers in the refrigerator or freezer, along with flour blends and mixes. Starches are best kept in airtight containers in the pantry.

Xanthan gum and guar gum (see page 21) should be refrigerated once the package is opened. I recommend dividing them in half, storing half in the freezer and half in the refrigerator, in airtight containers.

Quick-rising yeast should be stored in the refrigerator or freezer once opened; bring it to room temperature before using.

Always use clean storage containers that haven't been used for foods that might contain allergens, to avoid cross-contamination.

2.

Flour Blends *and* Baking Mixes

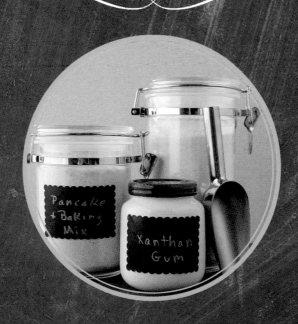

BASIC FLOUR BLEND ✧ BREAD FLOUR BLEND

PASTRY FLOUR BLEND ✧ PANCAKE AND BAKING MIX

One of the most important items in a well-stocked pantry is flour. If you are dealing with a wheat allergy, celiac disease, or non-celiac gluten sensitivity, you need to explore alternatives to traditional all-purpose wheat flour. Gluten-free grains are the place to start, and there are dozens to choose from. You will also learn about new ingredients—including starches and gums—to help compensate for the loss of gluten in wheat flour.

Gluten-free flours and flour blends vary dramatically in terms of taste, texture, and performance. Having performed extensive testing with different grains, different brands of flours, my own flour blends, and off-the-shelf flour blends, I can tell you that there is no such thing as a true "all-purpose" gluten-free flour blend. Flour blends described as such may actually be somewhat good for most baked goods, without excelling at any of them (or they may excel in select baked goods and flop in most others).

In this chapter I demystify flour blends, explain when to use which type of blend, and give substitution tips. With a few simple rules and blends you will be off to a great start stocking your own allergy-free pantry to enable you to make the best baked goods you can.

TAKING THE MYSTERY OUT OF FLOUR BLENDS

There are two rules to using flour blends successfully:

RULE #1: MEASURE FLOUR AND STARCHES BY WEIGHT RATHER THAN VOLUME.

The weight of the flour matters. Baking without dairy and eggs can be complicated, but neither ingredient is as critical to the outcome of your baked goods as getting the amount of flour right.

Gluten-free flour blends can weigh as much as 33 percent more than wheat flour. Products that appear to have the same ingredients (e.g., rice flour, tapioca starch, and potato starch) may have dramatically different weights. Even single-grain flours can vary dramatically in weight from brand to brand. For example, brown rice flour weighs between 30 and 40 grams per ¼ cup, and tapioca starch weighs between 32 and 40 grams per ¼ cup.

Some bakers fluff their flour, others sift, and others simply spoon from the bag. Some flour manufacturers sell their products in vacuum-sealed packages that are very densely packed, whereas others leave room in the packages for the flour to move around. Flours that are finely ground will settle more and weigh more per cup. All of these differences make it impossible to rely on volume measurements for flour.

The solution is simple: *measure flour by weight in grams (g)*.

I recommend a digital kitchen scale to measure flour (see tool tip on page 18). I recognize that it's different from what you may be used to, but once you start measuring by weight you will never look back. I feel so strongly about this that the recipes in this book lead with flour measurements by weight in this fashion:

128 grams (about 1 cup) Basic Flour Blend

Weighing eliminates possible error and gives you the most flexibility to substitute. The flour blends in this book weigh between 128 and 130 grams per cup. If you choose to substitute for the flours in these blends, do so by weight. For example, if a mix calls for 64 grams of sorghum and you'd rather use quinoa or gluten-free oat flour (both of which are usually lighter in weight), substitute 64 grams of the preferred flour, even if the volume measurement is more or less than the recipe suggests.

If you choose a brand of the same grain that is heavier or lighter than what my blend suggests, use the correct amount by weight.

RULE #2: WHENEVER POSSIBLE, MAINTAIN THE RATIO OF FLOUR TO STARCH.

At least one gluten-free grain must be combined with at least one starch to create a gluten-free flour blend. The starch helps with the texture of gluten-free baked goods and brings back some of the elasticity that gluten provides in traditional baked goods. The amount of starch in gluten-free flour blends varies from 30 to 70 percent, by weight. Yet starches are empty calories, containing no fiber or protein. I recommend only as much starch as you need for the type of baking you are doing.

Starches also behave differently than flours do—they absorb more liquid. If you substitute a flour blend that is 60 percent starch in a recipe that was developed to be made with 30 percent starch, you will most likely notice a gumminess or thickness in your baked goods. Conversely, if you try to make pizza dough with too little starch, the crust will crack because pizza dough needs more starch than muffin and cake batters do.

If you need to replace either the flours or starches in any of the flour blend recipes in this book, do so in equal proportions by weight. For example, if a recipe calls for 64 grams of brown rice flour and 32 grams of arrowroot starch, you may substitute 64 grams of sorghum flour and 32 grams of tapioca starch. My flour blends range from 20 percent starch for muffins and cakes (Basic Flour Blend, page 23) to 30 percent starch for breads (Bread Flour Blend, page 23) to 40 percent starch for pie crust and pastry (Pastry Flour Blend, page 24).

If you have just a single grain and a single starch available to you (due to allergies), please focus solely on the weight of the flours and the ratio of grain to starch (knowing that you will have to compromise on performance and taste). Most importantly, always choose grains that are safe for you and your family.

If *no* starches are safe for you, then (and only then) you may substitute flour for starch; however, in this case you should stick to recipes made with batters (such as muffins), and you may need to adjust the liquids. It's not possible or desirable to bake with starches alone.

FLOURS, STARCHES, AND GUMS

Wheat, barley, and rye contain gluten and must be avoided by those with a gluten-related illness such as celiac disease (for

tool tip

Digital kitchen scale

In order to measure flour you will need a digital scale. A simple, inexpensive scale that allows you to measure in grams and zero out the weight of a bowl is all you need.

simplicity I will refer to these illnesses collectively as "gluten allergy"). If you are allergic to gluten or wheat, you must avoid all forms of wheat, including spelt, kamut, and einkorn. If you are wheat-allergic but not sensitive to gluten, your physician may still advise you to avoid all of the gluten grains due to the potential for cross-contamination. For this reason, we will focus on gluten-free flours.

There are many gluten-free/soy-free/nut-free flours to choose from, and the options to combine them are seemingly endless. Typical gluten-free flour blends consist of rice flour (brown, white, or a combination) mixed with tapioca starch and potato starch. These generally do a decent job, but they only scratch the surface in terms of flavors that can be explored. Let's take a look at some of the flours we'll be using.

BASE FLOURS

There are a few gluten-free flours that work well as a starting point for a flour blend. These flours can easily be substituted for each other, in equal amounts by weight:

- **Millet flour**—Millet has a mild taste sometimes described as nutty. It pairs well with rice or sorghum flours.
- **Rice flours**—Rice flours are a staple in most gluten-free households. Brown rice flour contains a bit more protein and fiber than white rice flour. Sweet rice flour is not the same as rice flour (see page 20).
- **Sorghum flour**—This flour has more protein and fiber than brown rice and mixes well in flour blends. Sorghum is nearly tasteless and is considered

more easily digestible than other grains. Choose white (or "sweet" white) sorghum flour.

SPECIALTY FLOURS

There are a number of flours that can add taste or texture to gluten-free blends and are best used as an addition to flour blends rather than the base. They include:

- **Amaranth flour**—Amaranth is high in protein and fiber, and flour made from it lends a mild nutty taste to baked goods; it is best used in small amounts with either sorghum or rice flours.
- **Bean flours**—Bean flours can be made from garbanzo beans (also called chickpeas), fava beans, or a combination. Adding a small amount of bean flour to a blend will give bread a hearty taste.
- **Buckwheat flour**—I often combine a rice and sorghum blend with buckwheat for a light nutty taste that works well with chocolate.
- **Corn flour**—Corn flour provides a distinct taste and can be used alone or in combination with other flours. Masa harina (corn flour processed with lime) is ideal for making authentic-tasting Fajitas with Corn Tortillas (page 195).
- **Cornmeal**—Choose stone-ground cornmeal with a coarse grind. If you are allergic to corn and a recipe calls for dusting with cornmeal, substitute another flour used in the recipe's ingredients.
- **Oat flour**—Oat flour works fabulously in scones; always choose gluten-free

oat flour to avoid potential cross-contamination with wheat.

Potato flour—Potato flour is heavy and absorbs liquid quickly. It is especially useful in yeasted baked goods that need to hold a shape, such as Hamburger Buns (page 52). If you need to substitute for potato flour, your best bet is sweet rice flour or additional starch.

Sweet rice flour—While sweet rice is also known as glutinous rice, it doesn't actually contain gluten; the term describes the stickier quality of this rice. Although sweet rice flour is flour, it behaves a little bit like starch. A small amount of sweet rice flour works well in pastries and pizza crusts, which benefit from a chewier consistency. I recommend substituting it in small quantities for other flours, or using it to replace a starch that is not available to you due to allergies. I prefer to use superfine sweet rice flour.

As you select flours, keep in mind that not all brands will perform equally; I have witnessed dramatically different results from brand to brand of flours made from the same grain. Some flours are ground more finely than others, but a finer grain is not always best. I choose not to use superfine flours in my Basic Flour Blend (page 23) because they sometimes settle at the bottom of muffins or cakes, creating a gummy layer; however, their qualities shine in pastries and pie crusts. Conversely, flours that aren't ground finely enough can result in crumbly baked goods with a gritty taste.

Grinding Flour

FLOUR IS NOTHING more than grain that has been finely ground. If you are unable to find a safe source for allergen-free flours, one solution is to grind it at home. With the help of a high-speed food processor or blender, you can make flour from whole grains. If you plan to grind flours, consider purchasing the optional dry container that accompanies a blender you already own, or buy a blender that comes equipped with one.

Sorghum, millet, amaranth, buckwheat, quinoa, oat, and rice flours can all be made using this method:

1. Make sure the container for your high-speed blender or food processor is completely dry.

2. Measure the grains by weight. While the volume of the flour will change a bit as it becomes finer, the mass will not.

3. Use the high setting to grind the flour. The longer you grind, the finer the flour will become. Grind for thirty seconds at a time, stirring the flour in between, until the desired consistency is reached.

STARCHES

Starches are very important in gluten-free flour blends. At least one starch is required for a good mix, but the amount required varies tremendously depending on what you are baking. While choosing different flours will change the taste of your baked goods, your choice of starch will not. Starches are tasteless and, as noted earlier, void of significant nutritional value. Options include:

Arrowroot starch (also known as arrowroot flour)—Arrowroot starch comes from the root of Caribbean plants. While it's more expensive than tapioca starch, I find it blends extremely well and creates a smooth texture in baked goods.

Corn starch—Corn starch comes from the endosperm of the corn kernel and also substitutes well for other starches. Corn starch is known as corn flour in some parts of the world, but elsewhere, including the United States, corn starch and corn flour are different products (see page 19). I use the US terminology for both throughout this book.

Potato starch—Potato starch is very fine and usually used in combination with other starches in a flour blend; I don't recommend using it as the only starch in a flour blend unless necessitated due to allergies. Potato starch and potato flour are not the same; potato flour is the flour from a whole potato and tastes like potato (see page 20).

Tapioca starch (also known as tapioca flour)—Tapioca starch is favored by many gluten-free bakers; it is the standard in off-the-shelf gluten-free blends and can be found relatively inexpensively. Tapioca starch comes from the root of the cassava plant.

Any of these starches can be used to thicken soups, sauces, and puddings.

GUMS

Whereas starches help to replace some of the elasticity that gluten provides in traditional baking, gums are used to provide structure and help to hold baked goods together.

Xanthan gum—Xanthan gum is the most commonly used of the gums. My rule of thumb is ¼ teaspoon of xanthan gum per 128 to 130 grams (approximately 1 cup) of flour used. In baked goods that require more structure (such as bread) I sometimes use a little bit more.

Guar gum—If you are sensitive to xanthan gum, guar gum is the best replacement, but a bit more is needed. Use ½ teaspoon of guar gum per 128 to 130 grams (approximately 1 cup) of flour used. To substitute guar gum in a recipe that calls for xanthan gum, use double the amount.

Gums are very fine powders that become glue-like when they hit liquid. Always be sure to mix the gum into the dry ingredients extremely well before adding them to the liquid ingredients, to make sure it is distributed properly.

If you are sensitive to gums, you may omit them entirely, but your baked goods will crumble more than you might expect.

How to Measure Flour

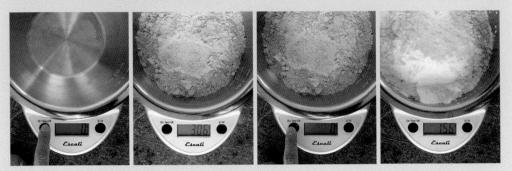

You should always weigh each flour and/or starch when you create a flour blend. When baking, weigh the flour blend and any additional flours or starches that the recipe calls for.

Regardless of how many flours and starches you are combining, all of them can be weighed together in one bowl as follows:

1. Power on your digital kitchen scale (see tool tip on page 18) and place a large mixing bowl on top of the scale. Set the unit to weigh in grams (g), rather than ounces or pounds. Weighing in grams provides the most precision.

2. Zero out the scale using the tare button; this may be the same as the power button. This step removes the weight of the mixing bowl.

3. Add the first flour to the mixing bowl until the correct gram weight for that flour is reached.

4. Hit the tare button again to set the scale back to zero and then add the next flour (in the same bowl) to the correct gram weight. Repeat this process until all of the flours and starches required for your blend are added.

5. Mix all of the flours and starches together extremely well.

FLOUR BLENDS

There are three flour blends you'll need when you begin stocking your pantry. My choices for the flours and starches in these blends are based on a combination of performance, taste, and nutritional value. I like to add higher-protein flours when possible and minimize the starch. You will also find a pancake and baking mix that even further simplifies a handful of everyday recipes.

I recommend that you mix flour blends in advance of baking in batches of 6 cups or less to ensure that they are well blended. Store the blends (and any opened packages of flour) in airtight containers in the refrigerator or freezer. The earliest expiration date on the flours you use to create your blend will determine how long you should keep the flour blend or baking mix.

Basic Flour Blend

MAKES 768 GRAMS (about 6 cups)
128 grams per cup, 80 percent flour,
20 percent starch

This simple flour blend can be used for muffins, quick breads, scones, cakes, and cookies that don't require a great deal of starch.

306 grams brown rice flour
306 grams sorghum flour
156 grams arrowroot starch

1. Measure each flour and the starch by weight in a large mixing bowl (see How to Measure Flour on page 22).

2. Mix the ingredients together extremely well. Store the blend in an airtight container in the refrigerator or freezer.

TO SUBSTITUTE

For a rice-free version, substitute millet flour for the brown rice flour. For a sorghum-free version, substitute white rice flour or millet flour for the sorghum flour.

Bread Flour Blend

MAKES 780 GRAMS (about 6 cups)
130 grams per cup; 70 percent flour,
30 percent starch

Bread and yeasted baked goods, such as Soft-Baked Pretzel Bites (page 206), require a flour blend with a bit more structure. The added starch and sweet rice flour help to give this blend a great texture. Millet adds a hearty taste.

256 grams brown rice flour
180 grams millet flour
120 grams superfine sweet rice flour
160 grams potato starch
64 grams arrowroot starch

1. Measure each flour and starch by weight in a large mixing bowl (see How to Measure Flour on page 22).

2. Mix the ingredients together extremely well. Store the blend in an airtight container in the refrigerator or freezer.

TO SUBSTITUTE

For a rice-free version, substitute sorghum flour for the brown rice flour and 60 grams of additional millet flour plus 60 grams of additional arrowroot starch for the sweet rice flour.

Pastry Flour Blend

MAKES 780 GRAMS (about 6 cups)
130 grams per cup; 60 percent flour,
40 percent starch

This flour blend is designed to be used with baked goods that require the ability to hold together while rolling and benefit from a finer, flakier crumb, such as pie crust.

288 grams brown rice flour

180 grams superfine sweet rice flour

192 grams tapioca starch

120 grams potato starch

1. Measure each flour and starch by weight in a large mixing bowl (see How to Measure Flour on page 22).

2. Mix the ingredients together extremely well. Store the blend in an airtight container in the refrigerator or freezer.

TO SUBSTITUTE

For a rice-free version, substitute sorghum flour for the brown rice flour and 90 grams of additional sorghum flour plus 90 grams of additional tapioca starch for the sweet rice flour.

Pancake and Baking Mix

MAKES 600 GRAMS (approximately 4½ cups)

Products described as pancake and baking mixes are nothing more than flour blends mixed with the other dry ingredients required to bake (including sugar, salt, and baking powder). Off-the-shelf versions usually have other ingredients—anticaking agents and preservatives—added as well.

This recipe builds on the Basic Flour Blend (page 23), adding ingredients to create an allergen-free version of Bisquick or other off-the-shelf pancake and baking mixes. It makes enough for two batches of Pancakes (page 120) or two batches of Biscuits (page 59).

512 grams (approximately 4 cups) Basic Flour Blend (page 23)

1 teaspoon xanthan gum

6 teaspoons baking powder

½ teaspoon salt

¼ cup plus 2 tablespoons (82 g) organic cane sugar

1. Mix all of the ingredients together extremely well in a large bowl.

2. Store the blend in an airtight container in the refrigerator or freezer.

OFF-THE-SHELF FLOUR BLENDS

You have the option to use off-the-shelf flour blends, should you prefer. I turn to them myself from time to time, and they are a great shortcut for those who are new to allergen-free baking. Nevertheless, some perform better and more consistently than others. My favorites include:

In place of Basic Flour Blend:
▶ King Arthur Flour Gluten-Free Whole Grain Flour Blend

In place of Bread Flour Blend:
▶ King Arthur Flour Gluten-Free Whole Grain Flour Blend
▶ Bob's Red Mill Gluten Free All Purpose Baking Flour

In place of Pastry Flour Blend (or for pizza crust):
▶ King Arthur Flour Gluten-Free Multi-Purpose Flour
▶ Authentic Foods Multi Blend Gluten-Free Flour

In place of Pancake and Baking Mix:
▶ Authentic Foods Pancake & Baking Mix
▶ King Arthur Flour Gluten-Free All-Purpose Baking Mix

When using an off-the-shelf blend, always use the correct amount by weight and check to see if a gum is included. If you choose a blend that already contains a gum (see page 21), leave out the gum called for in the recipe. Always check the ingredients label to ensure that the flour blend you choose is safe for your family, taking into consideration cross-contamination possibilities.

How To
SUBSTITUTE FLOURS

Always substitute by weight, maintaining the ratio of flour to starch (see page 18).

If you are using a recipe that was developed with wheat flour and you would like to use gluten-free flours: **Use 124 grams of a gluten-free flour blend for every cup of wheat flour called for.**

If you are using a recipe in this book with a modified flour blend (due to an allergy or for preference): **Refer to the weight (in grams) in the recipe and use the appropriate amount of flour by weight.**

If you are not allergic to wheat and you would like to use wheat flour with the recipes in this book: **Substitute equal amounts of wheat flour for the flour blends used, by weight. Omit the xanthan gum.**

If you are using a recipe in Learning to Bake Allergen-Free *and you would like to use one of the flour blends in this book:* **Choose a flour blend appropriate to the recipe and use 128 grams of your chosen blend per cup of flour called for in the recipe.**

If you are using a recipe found elsewhere and you would like to use one of the flour blends in this book: **If the recipe calls for flour by weight, substitute the correct amount of flour by weight. Otherwise, determine the weight of the flour blends suggested by the recipe. To do so you will need to know the brands of the flours used. Look at the nutrition label for that product to determine the grams per serving and the serving size. Calculate the grams per cup and adjust accordingly.**

3.

Non-Dairy
Milk *and* More

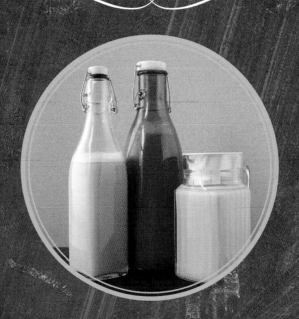

HEMP MILK ~ SUNFLOWER SEED MILK ~ RICE MILK ~ OAT MILK

WHIPPED COCONUT CREAM ~ HOMEMADE BUTTERY SPREAD

In recent years it has become much easier to find alternatives to cow's milk, soy milk, and nut milks. My grocery store now carries hemp milk, coconut milk beverage, and rice milk. Unsweetened versions as well as original (plain), vanilla, and often chocolate are available. You are welcome to use any versions of these off-the-shelf milks with your cereal or in your baking and cooking, if you find one that works with your food restrictions—I did for years.

The downsides to off-the-shelf non-dairy milks are that they are often manufactured in facilities that contain other allergens, they usually contain added preservatives and ingredients you might prefer to avoid, and they are expensive. A shelf-stable one-quart box of hemp milk costs about $4.50, whereas a single bag of shelled hemp seeds costing about $10.00 can produce four times the milk, and the price goes down if you buy the seeds in bulk.[*] More important, you can control how much you make at a time (thereby reducing waste), and you have complete control over the ingredients.

You may have guessed that I am going to teach you how to make non-dairy milk, and you are correct: recipes in this chapter include hemp, sunflower seed, rice, and oat milks, but I find that (without local access to coconuts) it's still easier and less expensive to buy coconut milk beverage at the grocery store. Nevertheless, see my tips on coconut milk on page 33.

NON-DAIRY MILK OPTIONS

Non-dairy and top-eight-allergen-free milks include rice, hemp, oat (make sure it's gluten-free), coconut, and sunflower. This list of off-the-shelf options keeps expanding as the market for these products grows. Until recently it wasn't possible to find sunflower seed milk, and the range of coconut milk beverages available has skyrocketed.

The formula for replacing cow's milk in recipes is a simple one-for-one substitution:

1 cup of cow's milk equals 1 cup of non-dairy milk.

Likewise, any non-dairy milk can be replaced for another, cup for cup, in recipes. I usually specify a non-dairy milk in recipes—most often hemp milk, for its superior nutritional qualities (it is naturally high in protein and omega essential fatty acids) and taste. I suggest coconut milk beverage in certain recipes, and sunflower seed milk in others. Nevertheless, if you are a tried-and-true rice milk lover, feel free to substitute rice milk (or another favorite) in equal amounts; indulge your own preferences or substitute to avoid allergens. If absolutely necessary, water can also be used (in equal amounts) as a substitute for milk in most baking recipes.

Each of the following recipes makes approximately 3 cups (720 ml) of milk; I find that working in small batches makes it easier to strain and store the milk. Use the milk immediately or refrigerate it in an airtight container. Without sugar or preservatives, most non-dairy milks will last for up to 3 weeks in the refrigerator. Non-dairy milk will separate (similar to orange juice); always shake it well before using.

---

[*] Cost will vary depending on ingredients and brands that are safe for you to use.

tool tip

Milk-Making Essentials

In addition to a blender or a food processor, a fine mesh strainer and a piece of cheesecloth are all the tools you need to make milk. Choose a double mesh strainer for the clearest milk.

Making Milk

Making milk is easier than you might think, but it does require advance planning. Follow these steps:

1. Let the ingredients for the milk (the seeds or grains plus water) soak in the container for your blender in the refrigerator for 8 to 12 hours or overnight.

2. Run the blender or food processor on high to puree the mixture for up to 1 minute (timing is dependent on the grain and the speed of your blender), until the seeds or grains are no longer visible.

3. Use a fine mesh strainer and/or cheesecloth (see tool tip on page 29) to strain the liquid into a bowl. To make the process easier, place a strainer underneath one or two pieces of cheesecloth to give it some structure. The pulp remaining from blending the seeds or grains into the water will be very fine.

4. If the drip of milk into the bowl slows, use a spoon to work the pulp away from the cloth. When there is a small amount of liquid left, pick up the cloth and gently massage the milk out with your hands, twisting and working your way from top to bottom. Discard the pasty claylike substance remaining in the cloth.

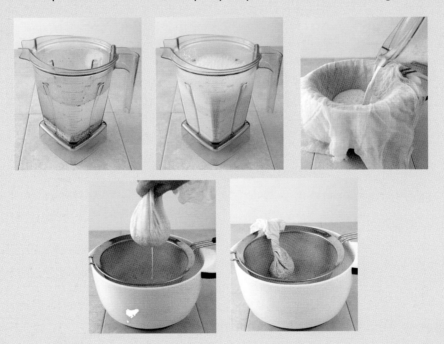

Hemp Milk

It's no secret that I love all things hemp. It was the first non-dairy milk that my son truly embraced, and even without a dairy allergy I now choose hemp milk for my own cereal. I find it very drinkable, even without added sweeteners. Hemp milk is easier to strain than some of the alternatives, which makes it a great recipe to start with when learning how to make milk. Homemade hemp milk is near white in color after straining, unlike the beige-colored milk you can purchase at the store.

½ cup (80 g) shelled hemp seeds
3 cups (720 ml) water

1. Combine the seeds and water and let them soak for 8 to 12 hours in the refrigerator.
2. Puree the seeds and water together in a high-speed blender or food processor until the seeds are no longer visible, about 1 minute.
3. Strain the seeds from the milk (see Making Milk on page 30). Use the milk immediately or refrigerate it in an airtight container for up to 3 weeks. Shake well before each use.

Sunflower Seed Milk

Sunflower seeds have a nutty taste. When you puree the seeds with water you will have great-tasting milk that adds flavor to cereal and granola or can be used in baking.

½ cup (72 g) shelled, unsalted, raw sunflower seeds
3 cups (720 ml) water

1. Rinse the seeds well.
2. Combine the seeds and water and let them soak for 8 to 12 hours in the refrigerator.
3. Puree the seeds and water together in a high-speed blender or food processor until the seeds are no longer visible, about 1 minute.
4. Strain the seeds from the milk (see Making Milk on page 30). Use the milk immediately or refrigerate it in an airtight container for up to 3 weeks. Shake well before each use.

Rice Milk

Rice milk is preferred by many due to its neutral taste. Whereas this recipe can be made with white rice, I find that brown rice works best. I prefer rice milk with a bit of sweetener; see the opposite page to learn what to add to this unsweetened version.

¾ cup (138 g) long grain brown rice
3 cups (720 ml) water

1. Combine the rice and water and let the mixture soak for 8 to 12 hours in the refrigerator.
2. Puree the rice and water together in a high-speed blender or food processor for 30 seconds. Overprocessed grains will make straining more difficult and result in milk with a grainy texture.
3. Strain the grains from the milk (see Making Milk on page 30). Use the milk immediately or refrigerate it in an airtight container for up to 3 weeks. Shake well before each use.

Oat Milk

Until recently oats were not an option for those allergic to wheat or gluten, due to the potential of cross-contamination with wheat. Now there are many sources of gluten-free oats, but gluten-free oat milk remains difficult to find. The solution is to make your own. Oats produce mildly sweet milk.

½ cup (48 g) gluten-free old-fashioned oats
3 cups (720 ml) water

1. Combine the oats and water and let the mixture soak for 8 to 12 hours in the refrigerator.
2. Puree the oats and water together with a high-speed blender or food processor until the oats are no longer visible, about 1 minute.
3. Strain the pulp from the milk (see Making Milk on page 30). Use the milk immediately or refrigerate it in an airtight container for up to 3 weeks. Shake well before each use.

FLAVORED MILKS

The recipes previously mentioned are for unsweetened milks. You have the option to add ingredients to vary the flavor and sugar content. Stir or blend in the added ingredients after straining the milk:

FOR VANILLA MILK

Add 1½ teaspoons Vanilla Extract (page 288) per 3 cups (720 ml) of milk.

FOR SWEETENED MILK

Add up to 1 tablespoon organic cane sugar or sweetener of choice (see page 8) per 3 cups (720 ml) of milk. This amount is roughly equivalent to the amount of sugar in off-the-shelf sweetened varieties of these milks.

FOR CHOCOLATE MILK

Add up to 2 tablespoons of Chocolate Syrup (page 292) per 3 cups (720 ml) of milk. Note that the chocolate syrup already contains sugar—there is no need to add more.

FOR BUTTERMILK TASTE

Add 1 tablespoon fresh lemon juice to 1 cup (240 ml) of milk.

COCONUT MILK PRODUCTS

It's important to note that whereas the Food Allergen Labeling Consumer Protection Act requires that coconut be labeled as a tree nut, it is not actually a nut. If a coconut product contains a warning that it contains tree nuts and you are allergic to tree nuts but not coconut, you should confirm with the company that there are no other nuts in the product. Nevertheless, it is possible to be allergic to coconut. Always follow your doctor's instructions.

As noted earlier, coconut milk is reasonably priced and available to most of us. If you choose coconut milk for drinking or baking, be sure to choose one labeled as a "beverage" rather than whole-fat coconut milk (that usually comes in a can), unless otherwise specified. Save the whole-fat canned varieties of coconut milk for making Whipped Coconut Cream (page 35). It should not be substituted when non-dairy milk is called for in a recipe.

You will also find some recipes in this book that call for coconut milk creamer, a relatively new product designed to replace the cream you might put in your coffee. It can be found in pint containers in the refrigerated section of the grocery store.

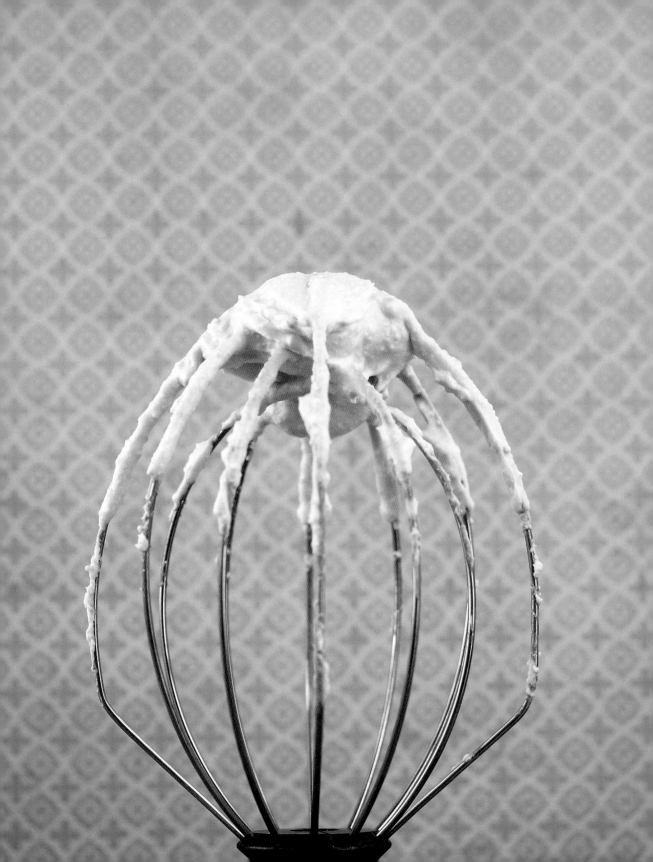

Whipped Coconut Cream

MAKES ABOUT 1½ CUPS (360 ML)

Who needs dairy whipped cream when you can have delicious whipped coconut cream? Serve it for dessert with fresh blueberries or with Chocolate Pudding (page 278). This recipe requires an electric mixer with a whipping attachment.

One 14-ounce (414 ml) can whole-fat coconut milk, refrigerated overnight

¼ cup (36 g) Powdered Sugar (page 286)

1. Chill a mixing bowl in the freezer for 2 hours.
2. Puncture the bottom of the refrigerated can of coconut milk and drain the liquid, reserving it for another use.
3. Open the can all the way and scoop the remaining cream into the chilled mixing bowl.
4. Use the whipping attachment on your mixer and mix on low for about 30 seconds to soften the cream. Turn the mixer up to high and whip for 20 to 30 seconds, until the cream is fluffy. Scrape down the sides of bowl, if needed.
5. Add the powdered sugar and whip for about 20 seconds longer. Refrigerate leftover cream in an airtight container and use it within 48 hours.

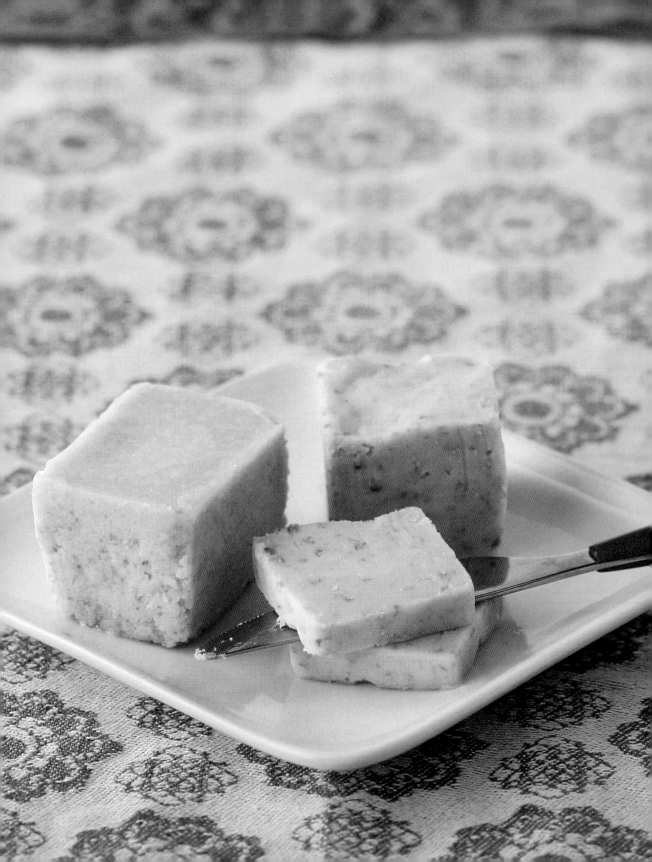

Homemade Buttery Spread

MAKES 1 CUP (240 ML)

*Y*ou may be delighted to discover that it is possible to make a non-dairy "buttery" spread at home. This spread is an emulsion created with oils and a tiny bit of protein. It's a tasty alternative to butter on your baked potatoes or English Muffins (page 131). I don't recommend using it to replace shortening in frosting or syrups, but it can be used (well chilled) when a cookie or pie crust recipe calls for shortening.

10 tablespoons coconut oil
3 tablespoons grapeseed oil
3 tablespoons organic canola oil
2 Flaxseed Eggs (page 42)
½ teaspoon fresh lemon juice
½ teaspoon salt

1. Heat the coconut oil in the microwave in a heat-resistant glass measuring cup with a pour spout, until just melted. Stir it to clarify and melt any tiny pieces, then let it sit to come back to near room temperature without solidifying.

2. Combine the grapeseed and canola oils in a separate measuring cup with a spout.

3. Combine the flaxseed eggs, lemon juice, and salt in a working glass or the container for your immersion blender, blender, or food processor. Pulse once or twice to combine the ingredients.

4. With the blender on a low continuous pulse, pour a few drops of the grapeseed and canola oil mixture into the container. The slower you pour, the better. The mix-ture will start to thicken as emulsification occurs. (See How to Create a Permanent Emulsion on page 94.)

5. Continue adding oil in a slow trickle, until all of the oil is incorporated. If the oil starts to pool on top of the mixture, slide your immersion blender up and down ½ inch or stop pouring until the oil combines.

6. Add the coconut oil last, in a slow drip, until the mixture is completely combined and creamy.

7. Spoon the buttery mixture into a silicone mold (see tool tip). Refrigerate for 4 to 5 hours, until completely set. Pop the buttery sticks out of the mold and transfer them to an airtight container. Refrigerate and use within 2 weeks.

TO SUBSTITUTE

Any oil can be substituted, in equal amounts, for the grapeseed and canola oils. I do not recommend substituting for the coconut oil; its ability to remain solid at room temperature is key to this recipe.

tool tip

Silicone mold

Use a silicone mold to shape buttery sticks and allow them to release easily after setting; choose a mold that holds 4 tablespoons (60 ml) per cavity (the equivalent of ½ stick of shortening).

How To
SUBSTITUTE MILKS

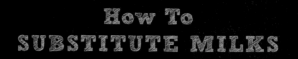

If you are using a recipe in this book that calls for a specific non-dairy milk and you would like to substitute another non-dairy milk (due to an allergy or preference): Substitute the preferred non-dairy milk in equal amounts, by volume.

If you are not allergic to dairy milk and would like to use it with recipes in this book: Substitute the dairy milk for the non-dairy milk in equal amounts, by volume.

If you would like to use an off-the-shelf non-dairy milk in lieu of the homemade versions in this book: Substitute the off-the-shelf milk in equal amounts, by volume (except for whole-fat coconut milk, see page 33).

If you would like to use one of the homemade milks in this book with recipes found in Learning to Bake Allergen-Free *or other cookbooks:* Substitute the homemade version in equal amounts, by volume.

4.

Replacing Eggs

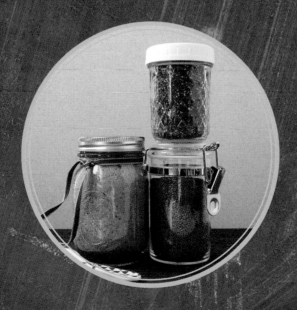

FLAXSEED EGGS ⌇ CHIA SEED EGGS ⌇ APPLESAUCE

Baking without eggs can be intimidating; there is no single ingredient that does everything an egg can do. Eggs provide texture and taste in traditional baked goods, harden when cooked, and provide leavening. Nevertheless, baking without eggs is possible, even when using gluten-free flours— the trick is to select the right candidate for the job.

Instead of eggs, most recipes in this book use preparations made from seeds or fruits. If you are unable to use seeds or fruits due to allergies, packaged egg replacers are the place to turn (see below).

SEEDS

Egg substitutes made from seeds have a consistency most like the consistency of traditional eggs prior to baking. One of my favorite choices is flaxseed gel or flaxseed "eggs"—flaxseed meal mixed with water. Chia seeds mixed with water provide a similar effect and can be substituted for flaxseed eggs in recipes.

While egg replacers made from seeds won't provide leavening, they do help to provide structure, give baked goods a moist crumb, and add some protein. I favor egg replacers made from seeds for muffins and breads. Flaxseed meal or chia seeds can also be added—in dry form—to baked goods to add nutrients and structure. If you are unable to use seeds due to an allergy and the recipe contains yeast, I recommend choosing a packaged egg replacer to replace the flaxseed eggs.

Mix Flaxseed Eggs or Chia Seed Eggs (page 42) a few minutes before you start your baking project as they require some time to gel.

FRUIT PUREE

Another option to replace eggs is fruit puree. Applesauce (page 45) is my first choice for fruit puree due to its mild flavor. While fruit puree doesn't provide the same binding effect as flaxseed eggs or chia seed eggs, it does provide some texture and taste. I favor fruit

purees as a substitute for eggs in recipes such as cookies and brownies.

Any fruit puree can be used to replace applesauce, in equal amounts. Mashed bananas, pear, mango, figs, even avocado can be used. If you choose a strong fruit, such as mango, the taste will be evident in your baked goods. If you are unable to use fruit, purees made from firm vegetables—winter squash, pumpkin, and sweet potato—can often be used to substitute for applesauce (and made using the same method).

PACKAGED EGG REPLACERS

Most egg-free baking recipes will call for more baking powder than traditional recipes, to assist with leavening. Packaged egg replacers can also be very useful in allergen-free baking. While some contain eggs and some contain dairy, others—including the popular Ener-G Egg Replacer—are free of the top eight food allergens.

Packaged egg replacers are actually amped-up baking powder and thus are best for leavening. I reserve packaged egg replacers for bread recipes that require a light texture, favoring the other options first, when possible. If you are unable to use seeds or fruit purees, use packaged egg replacers in place of either in recipes (but this will change the texture).

To make the equivalent of one egg, mix 1½ teaspoons of Ener-G Egg Replacer with 2 tablespoons warm water using a small whisk; let it sit for 2 minutes before using it in your recipe.

Make sure to check all of the ingredients for the packaged egg replacer you choose to ensure that it is safe for you and your family.

Flaxseed Eggs

MAKES THE EQUIVALENT OF 1 EGG
(just shy of ¼ cup/60 mL)

In addition to being used as an egg replacer, flaxseeds add fiber and omega-3 fatty acids to your food. Whole flaxseeds must be ground to be able to create flaxseed eggs and to be digested properly. Flaxseed Eggs can be made up to a few hours in advance of baking and stored in the refrigerator.

If you are allergic to flax, substitute Chia Seed Eggs (see below) for Flaxseed Eggs in recipes. If you are allergic to all seeds, choose a fruit puree (e.g., Applesauce, page 45) or Ener-G Egg Replacer (see page 41).

1 tablespoon ground flaxseeds (measured after grinding) or flaxseed meal

3 tablespoons warm water

1. Whisk the ingredients together in a small prep bowl with a small whisk or fork. Let it sit for 8 to 10 minutes to allow the flaxseed meal to absorb the water.

2. Whisk again to fully incorporate all of the water. Use it as directed in your recipe.

Chia Seed Eggs

MAKES THE EQUIVALENT OF 1 EGG
(just shy of ¼ cup/60 mL)

Chia seeds mixed with water provide a result that is similar to Flaxseed Eggs (see above). Chia seeds are another great source of fiber and omega-3 fatty acids. They should be used whole to make Chia Seed Eggs.

½ tablespoon chia seeds

3 tablespoons warm water

1. Whisk the ingredients together in a small prep bowl with a small whisk or fork. Let it sit for 8 to 10 minutes to allow the chia seeds to absorb the water.

2. Whisk again to fully incorporate all the water. Use it as directed in your recipe or in place of flaxseed eggs.

Grinding flaxseeds

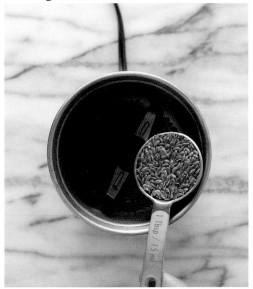 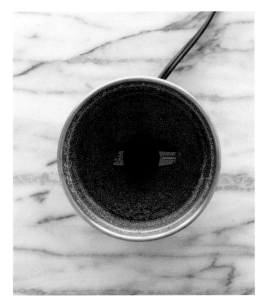

Making Flaxseed Eggs

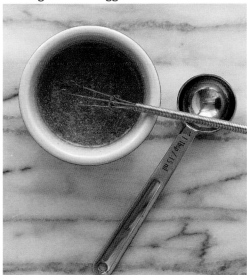 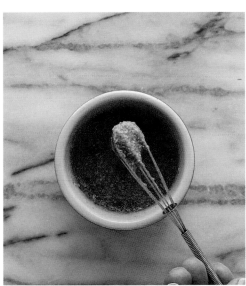

Seed grinder

Use a seed grinder (sometimes referred to as a spice and nut grinder) to grind whole flaxseeds into flaxseed meal. Avoid contamination by reserving this tool for grinding flaxseeds and other safe ingredients.

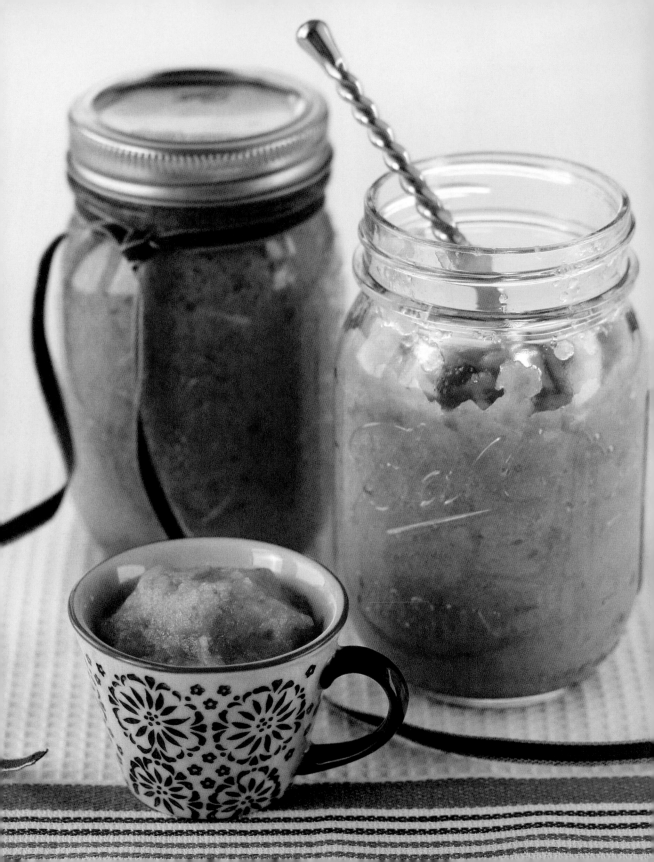

Applesauce

Making applesauce at home isn't much harder than boiling water. In the fall, when apples are plentiful, make large batches of applesauce and save it for use throughout the year. Store applesauce in the freezer in airtight, freezer-safe containers, or preserve it using a water bath. Applesauce can be used to replace eggs in recipes; use ¼ cup to replace one egg.

You may choose to substitute store-bought unsweetened applesauce when a recipe calls for applesauce; be sure to check the ingredients label.

10 medium apples (any kind), peeled, cored, and diced

About 6 cups (1440 ml) water

3 tablespoons fresh lemon juice (if canning)

1. Place the apples in a large pot and add just enough water to cover them. Bring it to a boil, uncovered, over medium-high heat.

2. If you are canning, start boiling the jars and follow the Steps for Canning on page 74.

3. Boil the apples for 10 to 15 minutes, until they are fork-tender. Take care not to let them get too mushy. Drain the water from the apples.

4. Place the apples in a food processor or blender and puree them until they are smooth.

5. If you are canning, add 1 tablespoon of lemon juice to each pint jar before adding the applesauce, leaving ½ inch (13 mm) of headspace (the amount of open space from the top of the filled jar to the lid), and process them in a water bath for 20 minutes (see page 74). Otherwise, let the applesauce cool completely before refrigerating or freezing in airtight containers. Refrigerate for up to 2 weeks. Freeze for up to six months; thaw in the refrigerator before using.

How To
SUBSTITUTE EGGS

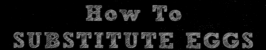

As a general rule *1 flaxseed egg, 1 chia seed egg, ¼ cup of apple-sauce (or another fruit puree), or 1 Ener-G egg (or other egg replacer, prepared according to package directions) can be substituted for each other;* however, each of these ingredients behaves differently. Although making substitutions in recipes is possible, if you substitute you may achieve different results.

If you have a recipe that was developed to use traditional eggs and you need to choose a replacement: **Choose flaxseed eggs, chia seed eggs, or applesauce for muffins, quick breads, cakes, and cookies. Choose flaxseed eggs, chia seed eggs, or Ener-G Egg Replacer for breads and pastry. Substitute in the amounts noted above.**

If you are using a recipe in this book that calls for flaxseed eggs and you are allergic to flaxseeds: **Replace the flaxseed eggs with chia seed eggs (unless you are allergic to chia seeds). Otherwise, choose applesauce (or another puree) when the recipe uses the Basic Flour Blend, and choose Ener-G Egg Replacer when the recipe uses the Bread or the Pastry Flour Blends.** *Exception:* **If a recipe uses flaxseed eggs as an emulsifying agent (e.g., Flaxseed Mayonnaise, page 99), the only substitutes that are viable are chia seed eggs or traditional eggs (if you are not allergic to them).**

If you are not allergic to eggs and would like to use traditional eggs instead of the egg replacers in the recipes in this book: **Use one egg for each flaxseed egg, Ener-G egg, or ¼ cup of applesauce (when it is being used to replace eggs) that the recipe calls for.**

An important caution about eggs: **While most allergies are to egg whites (the portion of the egg that contains the protein), it is impossible to completely separate the egg yolk from the egg white without risk of contamination. You must avoid** *both* **egg yolks and egg whites if you are allergic to eggs.**

5.

Breads, Rolls, *and* More

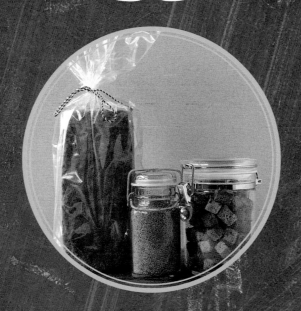

SANDWICH BREAD ~ HAMBURGER BUNS ~ CORNBREAD BITES

DINNER ROLLS ~ BISCUITS ~ BREADSTICKS ~ BREAD CRUMBS

CROUTONS ~ POLENTA CROUTONS ~ FLATBREAD

Bread is often the first thing missed when someone in the family can't eat wheat or gluten. Gluten-free options off the shelf and in restaurants sometimes contain dairy or soy, and nearly always contain eggs. Yet bread is on every food-allergy family's list of most coveted items, and when the kids go off to school—or you're packing yourself a lunch—it becomes a necessity.

USING QUICK-RISING YEAST AND PROOFING DOUGH

Gluten-free bread is easier to bake than traditional wheat bread; there is no need to let the dough rise twice, and there is no need for a long rise cycle using active dry yeast. Quick-rising yeast (sometimes called rapid-rise or fast-acting yeast) is the way to go.

Quick-rising yeast should be added in directly with the dry ingredients. Sugar or starch is needed in the recipe to ensure that the yeast does its job (yeast feeds on sugar and starches) and it's important not to overdo the salt—it interferes with the growth of yeast. When working with yeast, the balance of wet to dry ingredients is key. Note the desired texture in the recipe and add liquids to achieve the right consistency.

The most important step when working with quick-rising yeast is a short rise cycle: the dough needs to rise (or "proof") in a warm, humid spot; between 95°F and 100°F (35°C to 38°C) is ideal. This could be a warming zone on your stovetop that is set to low, an oven that has been warmed to the lowest setting and then turned off for a few minutes to cool down to below 120°F (48°C), or any warm spot in the house. A moist towel or plastic wrap sprinkled with a few drops of water and placed over the bread pan can help with the humidity if you are proofing on a stovetop (be sure not to let the plastic wrap touch the burner). If you are proofing in a heated and then cooled oven, fill an oven-safe container with water and place it on the lowest shelf of the oven during proofing.

Everything from the weather to the size of the baked goods you are making can affect how long your dough will take to rise. I have suggested proofing times within each recipe, but the trick is to catch the sweet spot where it has risen perfectly (just shy of double the original size) and before it starts to fall back. The total rise time for most yeasted recipes in this book will be between 30 and 40 minutes. Preheat the oven for baking 25 minutes into this cycle and continue to proof for another 5 to 10 minutes as the bread continues to rise. (If you are using your oven for proofing, be sure to take out the bread before preheating.) If you see pockmarks on the top of your bread or rolls, you have let them rise too long. Should this happen, pop them into the oven right away (you may notice some sinking during baking); adjust the timing in the future.

Digital thermometer

Bread is done when the internal temperature reaches 200°F to 205°F (93°C to 96°C). Look for a digital thermometer with a probe that can be inserted into the bread and left in the oven while you monitor the temperature without opening the oven door, or choose an instant-read thermometer. Check the temperature after the bread has baked for the minimum time specified in the recipe.

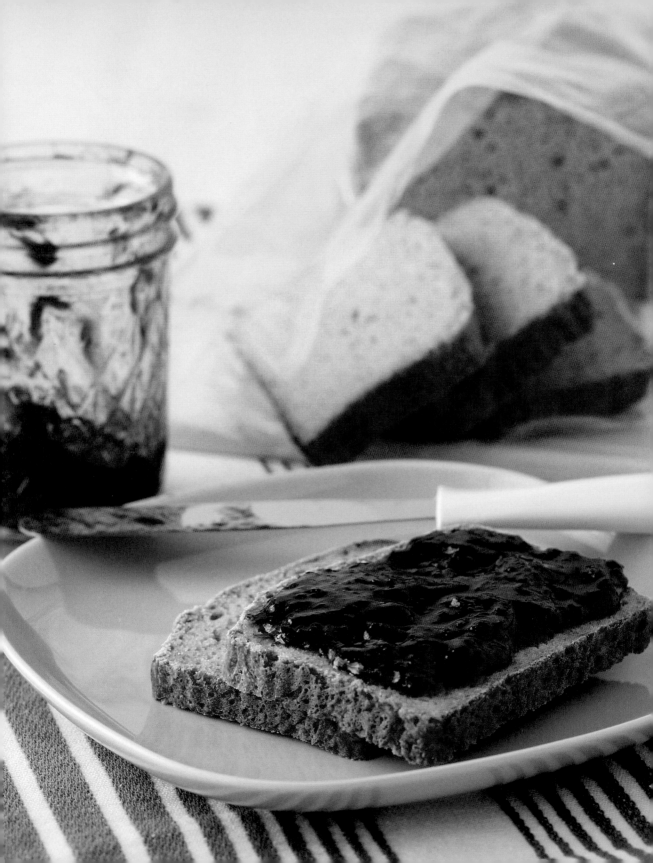

Sandwich Bread

Great sandwich bread without wheat, dairy, soy, or eggs? Yes, indeed! This is the bread you will turn to on a daily basis for making toast and packing lunch. Seek out a gluten-free bread pan that is a bit taller and narrower than a traditional bread pan to help the bread rise. Save some bread to make Bread Crumbs (page 63) and Croutons (page 64).

455 grams (about 3½ cups) Bread Flour Blend (page 23)

1 teaspoon xanthan gum

1 tablespoon quick-rising yeast

4 teaspoons baking powder

½ teaspoon salt

1 tablespoon organic cane sugar

⅓ cup (80 ml) grapeseed oil

3 Flaxseed Eggs (page 42)

1 cup (240 ml) warm water

1. Grease a 9 by 4 by 4-inch (23 by 10 by 10 cm) loaf pan.

2. Mix together the flour, xanthan gum, yeast, baking powder, salt, and sugar in a medium bowl.

3. Blend the oil, flaxseed eggs, and ¾ cup plus 2 tablespoons (210 ml) water together in a large bowl, using a mixer on medium speed, about 30 seconds.

4. Slowly add the dry ingredients to the wet ingredients and mix on medium-low speed until combined. Increase the speed to medium-high and beat for 2 minutes. Add up to 2 tablespoons of water as needed, ½ tablespoon at a time, until the dough is sticking to the sides of the mixing bowl.

5. Scoop the dough into the prepared loaf pan and spread it to the sides of the pan using a spatula, then use wet fingers to smooth the top.

6. Let the bread rise for 25 minutes in a warm, humid spot.

7. Preheat the oven to 375°F (190°C). Allow the bread to rise for another 5 to 10 minutes while the oven preheats. There should be about 1 inch (2.5 cm) clearance to the top of the pan when the dough is fully risen.

8. Bake for 37 to 41 minutes, until the internal temperature is 200°F to 205°F (93°C to 96°C). Remove the bread from the pan promptly and transfer it to a cooling rack. Let it cool completely before slicing.

TO FREEZE

Bread that you don't plan to use within 2 to 3 days can be frozen in airtight bags for up to 6 months. I recommend slicing before freezing so that you can remove slices as needed. Once frozen, bread will be best toasted.

TO SUBSTITUTE

If you are allergic to flaxseeds, substitute Chia Seed Eggs (page 42) or Ener-G Egg Replacer (see page 41) for the Flaxseed Eggs.

Hamburger Buns

The difference between hamburger buns and other breads is usually texture. This recipe adds potato flour (not to be confused with potato starch) to the Bread Flour Blend, and uses milk instead of water for a rich, moist crumb. But these buns aren't just for burgers; use them to make your favorite sandwiches too!

260 grams (about 2 cups) Bread Flour Blend (page 23)

90 grams (about ½ cup) potato flour

1 teaspoon xanthan gum

2¼ teaspoons quick-rising yeast

3 teaspoons baking powder

1 teaspoon salt

¼ cup (60 ml) sunflower oil

1 Flaxseed Egg (page 42)

1⅓ cups (320 ml) plus 2 tablespoons Hemp Milk (page 31) or non-dairy milk of choice, warmed to 100°F (38°C)

1. Line a large baking sheet with parchment paper.

2. Mix together the flours, xanthan gum, yeast, baking powder, and salt in a medium bowl.

3. Blend the oil, flaxseed egg, and 1⅓ cups (320 ml) of milk together in a large bowl, using a mixer on medium speed, about 30 seconds.

4. Slowly add the dry ingredients to the wet ingredients and mix on medium-low speed until combined. Increase the speed to medium-high and beat for 2 minutes. Add up to 2 tablespoons of milk as needed, ½ tablespoon at a time, until the dough is pliable and clustered in the center of the bowl.

5. Divide the dough into 8 equal sections. Use damp hands to form each section into a ball. Gently form each ball into a disk and place them on the prepared baking sheet, evenly spaced.

6. Let the buns rise for 25 minutes in a warm, humid spot.

7. Preheat the oven to 375°F (190°C). Allow the buns to rise for another 5 to 10 minutes while the oven preheats.

8. Bake for 21 to 23 minutes, until the internal temperature is 200°F to 205°F (93°C to 96°C). Let the buns cool completely before slicing.

TO FREEZE

Buns that you don't plan to eat within 2 to 3 days can be frozen in an airtight container for up to 6 months. I recommend slicing before freezing. Once frozen, buns will be best toasted.

TO SUBSTITUTE

If you are allergic to flaxseeds, substitute Chia Seed Egg (page 42) or Ener-G Egg Replacer (see page 41) for the Flaxseed Egg.

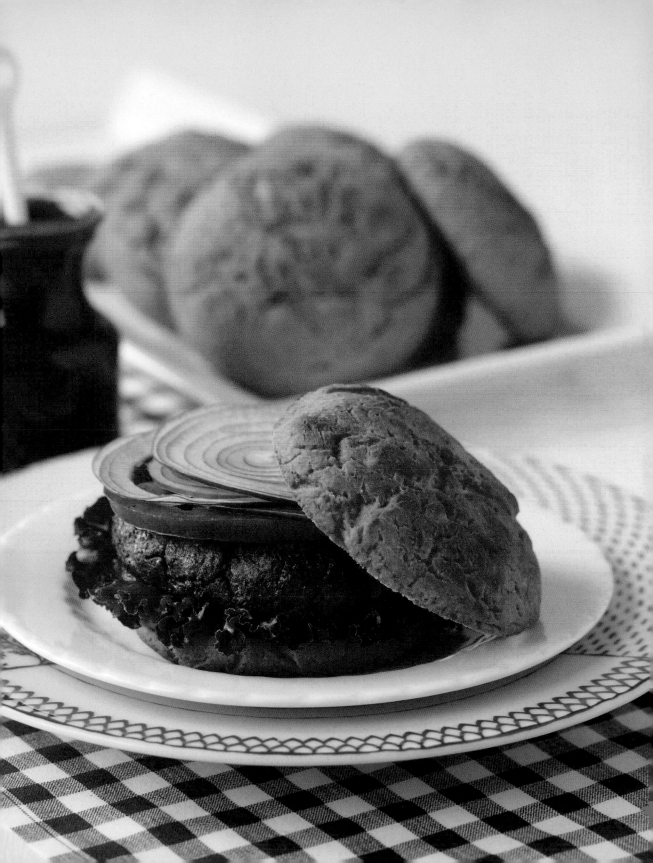

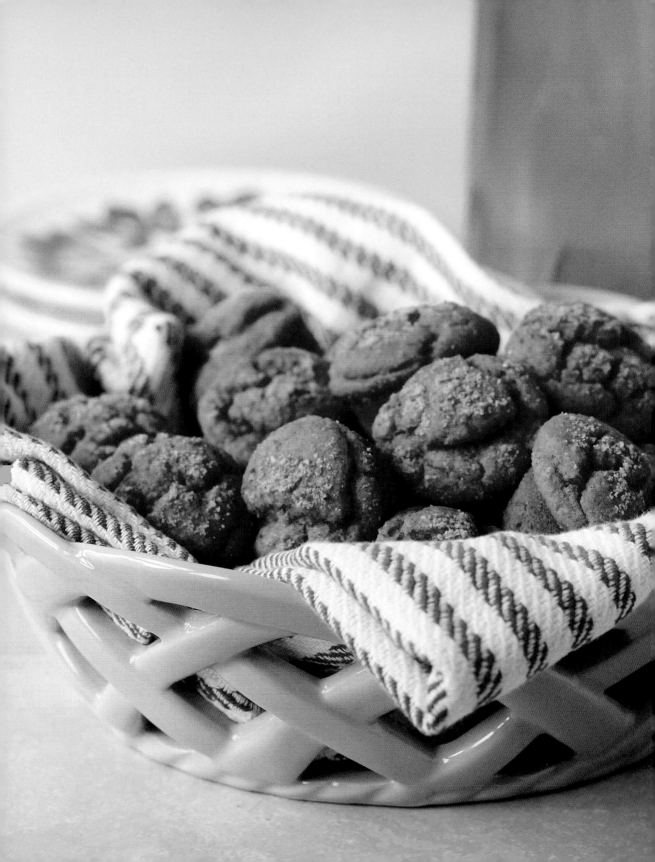

Cornbread Bites

Cornbread was first made by Native Americans and thus might be considered the national bread of North America. It's no wonder we love it so much! This low-sugar, bite-sized version is perfect for stashing in a lunch box. Both little hands and big hands are going to love them!

128 grams (about 1 cup) Basic Flour Blend (page 23)

116 grams (about 1 cup) corn flour

¼ cup (33 g) plus 1 tablespoon cornmeal

½ teaspoon xanthan gum

3 teaspoons baking powder

½ teaspoon salt

¼ cup (60 ml) agave nectar

1 cup (240 ml) coconut milk beverage or non-dairy milk of choice

2 teaspoons fresh lemon juice

½ cup (120 ml) sunflower oil

½ cup (120 g) Applesauce (page 45)

1. Preheat the oven to 350°F (180°C). Grease the cups of a 24-cup mini-muffin pan.
2. Combine the flours, ¼ cup (33 g) cornmeal, xanthan gum, baking powder, and salt in a medium bowl.
3. Blend the agave nectar, milk, lemon juice, oil, and applesauce together in a large bowl, using a mixer on medium speed or by hand with a spoon, about 1 minute.
4. Add the dry ingredients to the wet ingredients and mix for 1 to 2 minutes, until completely combined.
5. Spoon the batter evenly into the cups of the prepared mini-muffin pan. Sprinkle the tops of the muffins with the remaining cornmeal. Bake for 18 to 20 minutes, until the tops are golden and a toothpick inserted comes out clean.

TO FREEZE

Muffins that won't be eaten within 2 to 3 days can be frozen in an airtight container for up to 6 months. Thaw and reheat at 325°F (165°C) for 6 to 7 minutes.

Dinner Rolls

For years I have been searching for the perfect dinner roll. I have found some great gluten-free and dairy-free options, but egg-free? That's a challenge most gluten-free food vendors haven't yet stepped up to. This recipe has the perfect mix of flours to create a great-tasting dinner roll that can be topped with Homemade Buttery Spread (page 37) or dipped in olive oil. These can be made as pull-apart rolls in a baking dish or stand-alone on a baking sheet.

325 grams (page 23) Bread Flour Blend (about 2½ cups)

60 grams (about ½ cup) superfine sweet rice flour

34 grams (about 3 tablespoons) potato flour

1 teaspoon xanthan gum

2¼ teaspoons quick-rising yeast

1 tablespoon organic cane sugar

3 teaspoons baking powder

1 teaspoon salt

¼ cup plus 2 tablespoons (90 ml) grapeseed oil

2 Flaxseed Eggs (page 42)

1 tablespoon apple cider vinegar

1 cup (240 ml) plus 2 tablespoons warm water

1. Grease a 7 by 9-inch (18 by 23 cm) baking dish (for pull-apart rolls) or line a large baking sheet with parchment paper (for individual rolls).

2. Combine the flours, xanthan gum, yeast, sugar, baking powder, and salt in a medium bowl.

3. Blend the oil, flaxseed eggs, vinegar, and 1 cup (240 ml) of water together in a large bowl, using a mixer on medium speed, about 1 minute.

4. Slowly add the dry ingredients to the wet ingredients and mix on medium-low speed until combined. Increase the speed to medium-high and beat for 2 minutes.

Add up to 2 tablespoons of water as needed, ½ tablespoon at a time, until the dough is thick and pliable.

5. Divide the dough into 12 equal sections. Use damp hands to form each section into a ball and smooth the tops. Place them in the baking dish in 3 rows of 4 rolls each, with the sides touching (to make pull-apart rolls), or on the baking sheet with space in between (to make individual rolls).

6. Let the rolls rise for 25 minutes in a warm, humid spot.

7. Preheat the oven to 375°F (190°C). Allow the rolls to rise for another 5 to 10 minutes while the oven preheats.

8. Bake for 24 to 25 minutes if using a baking dish or 19 to 20 minutes if using a baking sheet, until the internal temperature is 200°F to 205°F (93°C to 96°C).

TO FREEZE

Rolls that you don't plan to use within 2 to 3 days can be frozen in an airtight container for up to 6 months. Thaw and reheat at 325°F (165°C) for 8 to 10 minutes.

TO SUBSTITUTE

If you are allergic to flaxseeds, substitute Chia Seed Eggs (page 42) or Ener-G Egg Replacer (see page 41) for the Flaxseed Eggs.

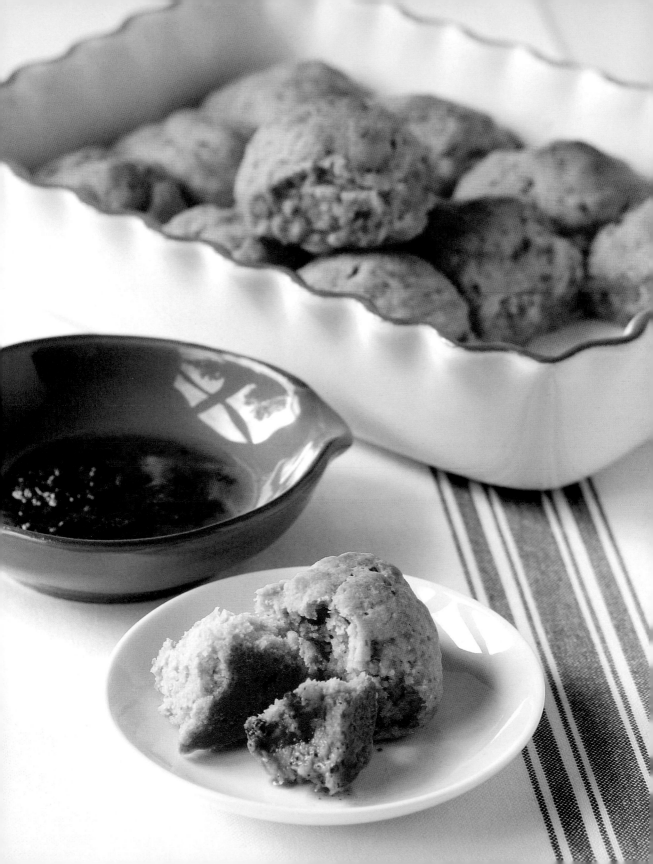

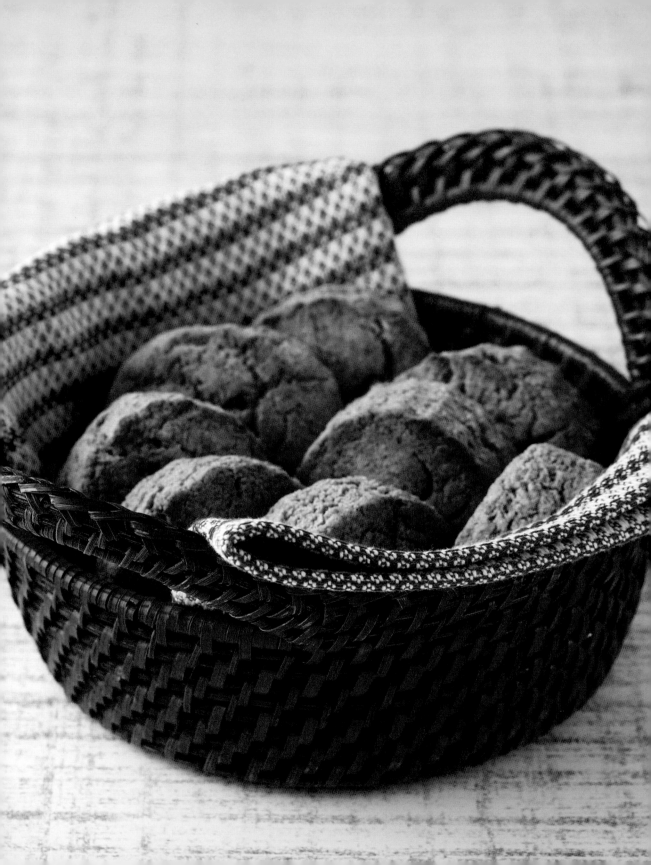

Biscuits

Whereas rolls usually require yeast, biscuits are more akin to a muffin or a scone—no yeast is required. If you need to avoid yeast or you are searching for the quickest bread to make for dinner, these versatile biscuits made with Pancake and Baking Mix (page 24) will do the trick. They can be made—start to finish—in just 20 minutes.

2 tablespoons light olive oil

⅔ cup (160 ml) Hemp Milk (page 31) or non-dairy milk of choice

266 grams (about 2 cups) Pancake and Baking Mix (page 24), plus up to 2 more tablespoons for dusting

1. Preheat the oven to 400°F (200°C). Line a large baking sheet with parchment paper.
2. Combine the oil and milk in a large mixing bowl. Stir in 266 grams of the baking mix and blend by hand until a thick batter forms into a ball.
3. Sprinkle a light dusting of baking mix on a smooth prep surface and scoop the dough on top. Use more flour as needed to keep the dough from sticking.
4. Use your hands to gently pat the dough into a disk about ½ inch (13 mm) thick. Use a knife or biscuit cutter to cut eight 2-inch (5 cm) round biscuits and place them on the prepared baking sheet.
5. Bake for 12 to 13 minutes, until a toothpick inserted comes out clean.

TO FREEZE

Biscuits that won't be eaten within 2 to 3 days can be frozen in an airtight container for up to 6 months. Thaw and reheat at 325°F (165°C) for 7 to 8 minutes.

Breadsticks

Potato flour gives these breadsticks a pull-apart texture that have made them a family favorite. They are soft, yummy, and garlicky (if you choose)—the perfect complement to your favorite pasta dish.

260 grams (about 2 cups) Bread Flour Blend (page 23)

45 grams (about ¼ cup) potato flour

1 teaspoon xanthan gum

2¼ teaspoons quick-rising yeast

2 teaspoons baking powder

½ teaspoon salt

1½ teaspoons Ener-G Egg Replacer mixed with 2 tablespoons warm water

¼ cup (60 ml) plus 1 tablespoon light olive oil

1 cup (240 ml) plus 1 tablespoon warm water

1 tablespoon garlic powder, optional

1. Line a large baking sheet with parchment paper.
2. Mix together the flours, xanthan gum, yeast, baking powder, and salt in a medium bowl.
3. Blend the egg replacer, ¼ cup (60 ml) of the oil, and 1 cup (240 ml) of the warm water together in a large bowl, using a mixer on medium speed, for 30 seconds.
4. Slowly add the dry ingredients to the wet ingredients and mix on medium-low speed until combined. Increase the speed to medium-high and beat for 2 minutes. Add up to 1 more tablespoon of warm water as needed, ½ tablespoon at a time, until the dough is thick and pliable.
5. Divide the dough into 8 equal sections. Form each section into a ball, then roll it between your palms or against a smooth prep surface to create a stick about ¾ inch (19 mm) thick and 7 to 8 inches (19 to 20 cm) long. Place the breadsticks on the prepared baking sheet.
6. Let the breadsticks rise for 25 minutes in a warm, humid spot.
7. Preheat the oven to 375°F (190°C). Allow the breadsticks to rise for another 5 to 10 minutes while the oven preheats.
8. Brush the tops of the breadsticks with the remaining oil and sprinkle with garlic powder, if desired. Bake for 15 to 16 minutes, until lightly browned and the internal temperature is 200°F to 205°F (93°C to 96°C).

TO FREEZE

Breadsticks that you don't plan to use within 2 to 3 days can be frozen in airtight containers for up to 6 months. Thaw and reheat at 325°F (165°C) for 7 to 8 minutes.

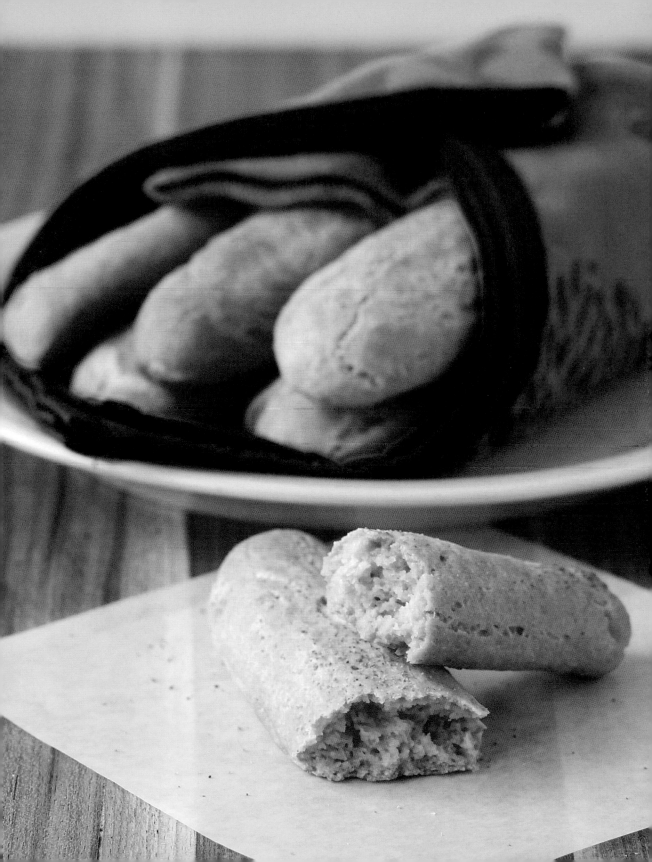

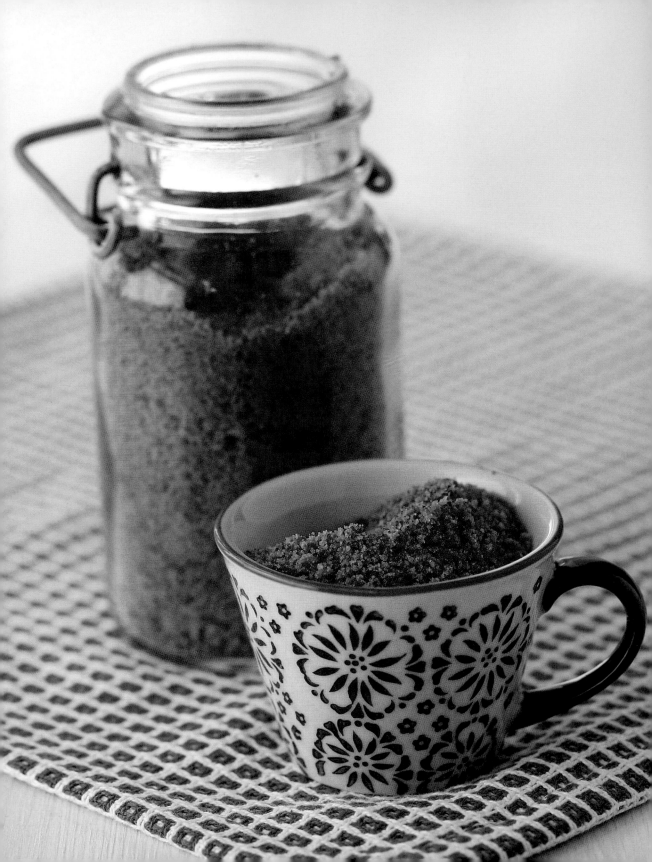

Bread Crumbs

Why buy expensive gluten-free bread crumbs when you can make them easily at home? With just a few slices of bread you can craft your own bread crumbs to make Meatloaf (page 196) or Chicken Tenders (page 191). Add seasonings to suit your taste, or leave them unseasoned. Due to their moisture content, I don't recommend substituting the other breads and rolls from this book for the Sandwich Bread in the recipe, but you may substitute a safe, off-the-shelf sandwich bread.

2 cups (140 g) Sandwich Bread (page 51), cut into uniform cubes (about ¾ inch/19 mm)

¼ teaspoon salt

OPTIONAL SEASONINGS:
¼ teaspoon garlic powder
½ teaspoon dried parsley
½ teaspoon dried basil
½ teaspoon dried oregano

1. Preheat the oven to 325°F (165°C). Line a large baking sheet with parchment paper.

2. Spread the bread cubes on a baking sheet. Bake for 10 minutes, flip them over, and bake for 8 to 10 minutes longer. Baking will dry out the bread. Let the bread cubes cool completely (at least 15 minutes).

3. Place the dried bread cubes, salt, and optional seasonings in a blender or food processor and give it a few pulses until you reach the desired grain. It's best not to overprocess them.

4. Store unseasoned bread crumbs in the refrigerator in an airtight container for up to 1 month; seasoned bread crumbs should be used within 1 week.

TO FREEZE

Freeze unseasoned bread crumbs for up to 6 months in an airtight container. Thaw at room temperature in the refrigerator.

VARIATIONS

If you don't have bread handy when you need bread crumbs, they can be made using a variety of dried cereals, including gluten-free corn flakes and gluten-free crisped rice. Choose an unsweetened cereal with no added ingredients and skip ahead to step 3.

Croutons

I'm tired of the answer to croutons being "Just leave them off." At home it's simple to use your favorite off-the-shelf bread or Sandwich Bread (page 51) to create croutons for your soups and salads. Vary the seasonings to suit your taste and avoid allergens; leave off the olive oil and seasonings if you plan to freeze them.

2 cups (140 g) of Sandwich Bread (page 51), cut into uniform cubes (about ½ inch/13 mm or desired size)

OPTIONAL TOPPINGS:
Olive oil in a spray mister
⅛ teaspoon salt
½ tablespoon dried parsley

1. Line a large baking sheet with parchment paper. Preheat the broiler (use the normal broiler setting, or high if your oven has a high and a low setting).
2. Spread the bread cubes on the lined baking sheet, without overlap.
3. Lightly spray the bread cubes with olive oil. Sprinkle the seasonings over the bread cubes, if desired.
4. Place the baking sheet on the second shelf below the broiler. Broil for 1½ to 2½ minutes (depending on the size of your croutons and how quickly your broiler cooks). Watch them closely so they don't burn.
5. Remove the croutons from the oven, flip them over, and broil for another 1 to 2 minutes. Your croutons should be lightly browned, slightly crunchy, and ready for your salad.

TO FREEZE

These are best when used the same day, but if you plan to keep croutons longer, leave off the olive oil and seasonings; freeze them in an airtight container for up to 6 months. Thaw at room temperature, then reheat at 400°F (200°C) for 6 to 7 minutes.

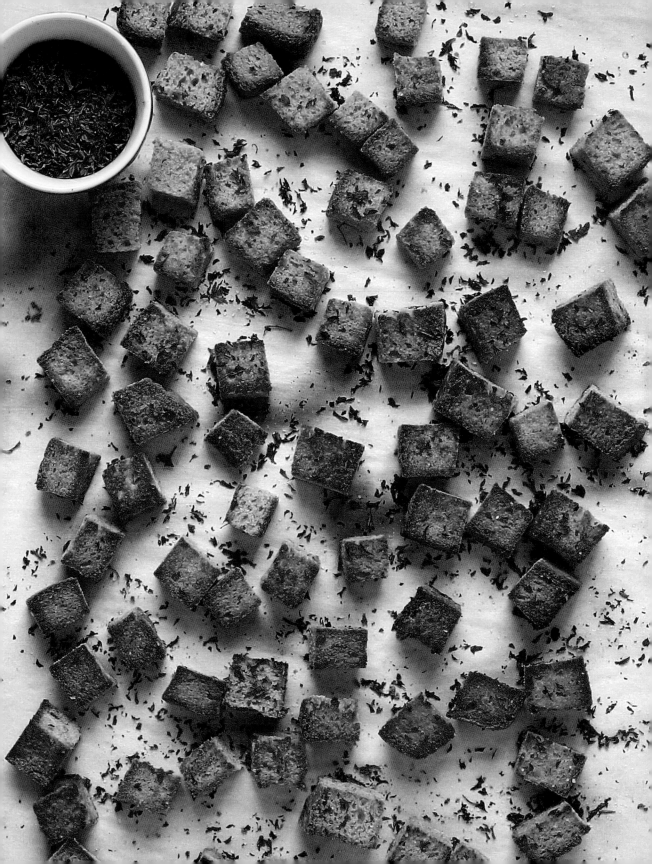

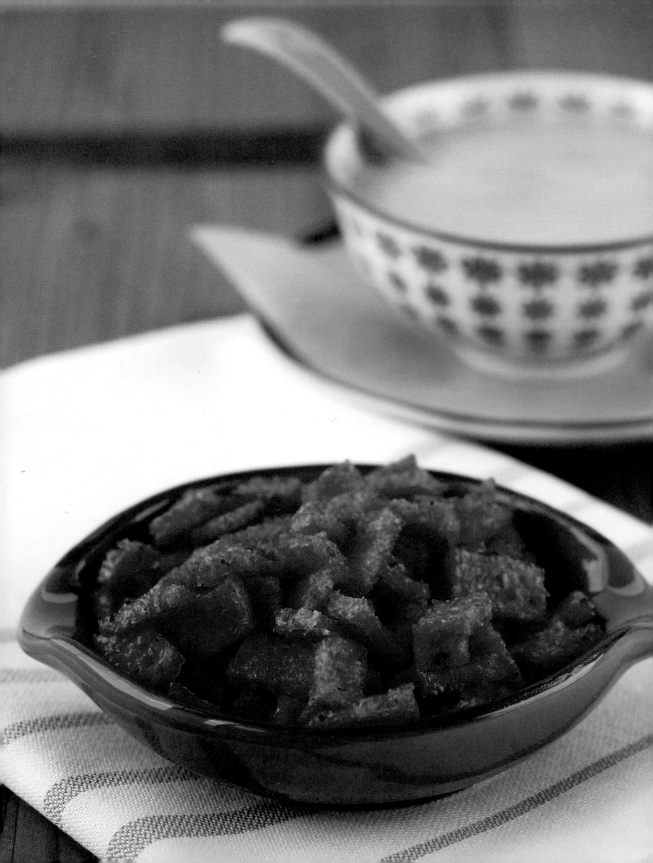

Polenta Croutons

I remember the day I discovered polenta croutons at one of my favorite restaurants. I was able to enjoy croutons that are not only gluten-free but also dairy-free and egg-free. Those crunchy croutons, made from polenta, rocked my world and inspired this recipe.

½ batch Polenta (page 140), chilled for at least 4 hours

1. Preheat the oven to 450°F (230°C). Line a large baking sheet with parchment paper.
2. Use a flat knife to loosen the polenta from the edges of the container it was chilled in and transfer it to a cutting board. Use a paper towel to blot excess moisture from the polenta.
3. Use a sharp knife to create long sticks of polenta about ½ inch (13 mm) thick, then slice each of the sticks into croutons about ⅛ inch (3 mm) wide. Place the croutons in a single layer on the baking sheet.
4. Bake for 20 to 22 minutes, until crispy and lightly browned.

TO FREEZE

Croutons not used within 2 days can be frozen in an airtight container for up to 6 months. Reheat from frozen at 375°F (190°C) for 7 to 8 minutes.

Flatbread

This multipurpose bread can be topped for a quick pizza crust, used as pita pockets, or scored and baked to make Pita Chips (page 231). It can also be served with Hummus (page 213) or added to a gluten-free breadbasket. Cook flatbreads on the stovetop in a dry skillet; they will brown nicely while staying moist inside.

If you wish to use these as pita pockets, I suggest making 4 larger (8-inch/20 cm round) breads. Let them cool completely before carefully scoring the centers with a sharp knife.

260 grams (about 2 cups) Bread Flour Blend (page 23)

½ teaspoon xanthan gum

2¼ teaspoons quick-rising yeast

½ tablespoon organic cane sugar

1 teaspoon baking powder

½ teaspoon salt

1 Flaxseed Egg (page 42)

1 tablespoon light olive oil

½ cup (120 ml) plus 1 tablespoon warm water

Up to 4 tablespoons additional flour for dusting

1. Combine the flour, xanthan gum, yeast, sugar, baking powder, and salt in a medium bowl. Set it aside.
2. Blend the flaxseed egg, oil, and ½ cup (120 ml) of the warm water together in a large bowl, using a mixer on medium speed, for 30 seconds.
3. Add the dry ingredients to the wet ingredients and mix on medium-low speed until combined. Increase the speed to medium-high and beat for 2 minutes. Add up to 1 more tablespoon of the water as needed, ½ tablespoon at a time, until the dough is pulling away from the sides of the bowl.
4. Line a large baking sheet with parchment paper. Divide the dough into 8 portions.

Use damp hands to roll the portions into balls and place them on the baking sheet. The trick to round edges for the bread is to keep the outer layer of the balls moist while rising. Let the dough rise for 25 minutes in a warm, humid spot.

5. Preheat a large skillet on medium-high heat.
6. Spread a thin layer of flour on a smooth prep surface or another piece of parchment paper. Use a small rolling pin with light pressure to create 5-inch (13 cm) rounds from the balls. Use extra flour as needed to avoid sticking.
7. Lower the skillet heat to medium. Grill each flatbread for about 1 minute per side, being careful not to let them burn.

TO FREEZE

Flatbreads not used within 2 to 3 days can be frozen in an airtight container for up to 6 months. Thaw them at room temperature.

TO SUBSTITUTE

If you are allergic to flaxseeds, substitute a Chia Seed Egg (page 42) or Ener-G Egg Replacer (see page 41) for the Flaxseed Egg.

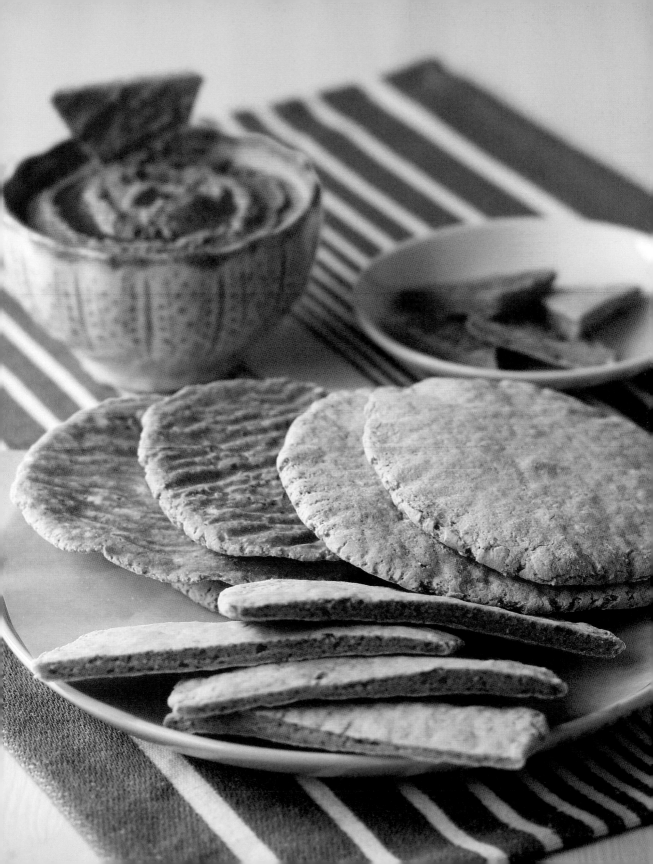

6.

Butters and Jams

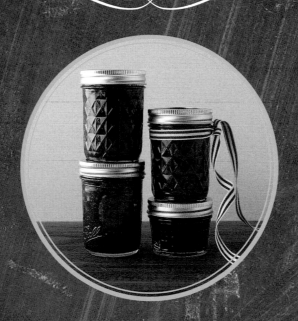

SUNFLOWER SEED BUTTER ✑ CHOCOLATE SUNFLOWER BUTTER

APPLE BUTTER ✑ STRAWBERRY JAM ✑ FIGGY PEAR JAM

HONEY BLUEBERRY ZEST JAM ✑ CHERRY VANILLA JAM

I grew up on peanut butter and jam sandwiches (heavy on the jam, please). And, like most parents, I sent my kids to school with those same sandwiches on occasion—until we learned that my son was allergic to peanuts. But he can still enjoy a healthy version of those sandwiches today.

Sunflower seed butters and apple butter are satisfying and quite easy to make at home. Making jam is a fabulous way to save a little bit (or a lot) of summer's fresh fruit for later in the year, and it's a great way to save money if you buy fruit locally, in season, and on sale. When I discovered how much fun it is to make my own jams and butters I stopped buying them from the store completely. Always be sure to buy fresh, just-ripe fruit if you plan to preserve your jams.

Making butters and jams at home also gives you control over the ingredients. Allergic to lemons? Leave out the lemon juice (only in high-acid fruit jams) or substitute another acid (see page 10). Want a lower-sugar version? The choice is yours. Keep in mind that the sugar and the lemon juice act as preservatives, allowing you to keep it on the shelf or in the refrigerator longer.

CANNING JAM AND OTHER HIGH-ACID FOODS

Canning is the process of cooking food and sealing it in sterile jars. The biggest risk in canning or preserving is not mold or yeast—or even cross-contamination—it's botulism. The bacteria that cause botulism survive harmlessly on the skins of fruits and vegetables; in the absence of air they can spread and create a deadly toxin; boiling the filled jars in a water bath weakens the bacteria, making the food safe to consume at a later date.

As long as the food being preserved has a pH level of 4.6 or lower, it can be processed in a water bath; vegetables and meats must be processed using pressure canning (a technique not covered here). The pantry items in this book that you might choose to can include jams, applesauce, apple butter, tomato sauce, ketchup, and pickles. All can be preserved using the water bath method described on page 74.

Keep in mind that this text is not a comprehensive guide on canning. Refer to the U.S. Department of Agriculture's *Complete Guide to Home Canning and Preserving* to learn more and ensure that you are canning safely. The USDA's proper canning practices include:

▶ Carefully selecting and washing fresh food

▶ Peeling some fresh foods

▶ Hot packing many foods

▶ Adding acids (lemon juice or vinegar) to some foods

▶ Using acceptable jars and self-sealing lids

▶ Processing jars in a boiling water or pressure canner for the correct period of time*

Always use fresh foods and wash them thoroughly. Remove any spoiled fruit or bad spots. Acids must be added to the Figgy Pear Jam (page 85), Marinara Sauce (page 178), and Ketchup (page 95) recipes in this book to ensure that the proper pH level is reached. Tomatoes must be peeled when preserving Marinara Sauce or Ketchup.

---

* U.S. Department of Agriculture, *Complete Guide to Home Canning and Preserving*, Second Revised Edition (Mineola, NY: Dover Publications, 1999), 1–5.

Pickles (page 209) must be processed with a high-acid brine.

Be sure to use jars and lids that are in good condition. Inspect them for cracks and chips. Always use two-part lids consisting of a sealing lid and a ring. The jars and rings can be reused. Always use a new sealing lid.

Steps for Canning

If you plan to preserve food using a water bath, you must follow these steps while the food is being prepared:

1. Place the canning jars in a large pot with a rack so that the jars are not touching the bottom of the pan. Fill the pot with water to at least 1 inch (2.5 cm) above the jars. Cover the pot and boil the jars. Boiling the jars serves two purposes: to sanitize the jars and to prepare them to accept hot food. The jars must be boiled for at least 10 minutes; start the timer after the pot reaches a full rolling boil.

2. Soften the lids in a small saucepan filled with enough water to cover the lids, over low heat. Always use two-part lids with new seals. The lids need to be softened so that they can create a proper vacuum seal.

3. When the food is ready, remove the jars from the boiling water using a jar lifter. Carefully tip the jars to release the water into the pot. You may need to remove some water from the pot to avoid overflowing once the jars are filled. Place the jars on a heat-resistant surface. Remove the lids from the saucepan with tongs or a lid lifter and have them ready to go.

4. Spoon the food into the hot, sanitized jars using a wide-mouth funnel. Leave ¼ inch (6.5 mm, for most jams) to ½ inch (13 mm) of headspace (the amount of open space from the top of the filled jar to the lid), following the recipe. Wipe the rims of the jars so that a proper seal can form.

5. Place the lids on top of the jars and secure them with the rings (just lightly tightened). Use an oven mitt to hold the hot jars as you do this. Do not over-tighten the lids; the jam or sauce needs to vent during processing.

6. Return the jars to the boiling water using a jar lifter. Cover the pot and boil for the amount of time specified in the recipe. This will vary from 10 to 35 minutes for the recipes in this book. Processing for the correct amount of time is extremely important for safety.

7. Uncover the pot and let the jars sit in the pot for 5 minutes. Use a jar lifter to remove the jars from the water and place them on a heat-resistant surface to cool. Do not tip the jars. Do not tighten the rings. The rings are there to allow

the lids to stay put during processing. Once removed from the water bath a vacuum seal will occur. You know you are successful when you hear the lids of the jars pop as that vacuum occurs.

8. Let the jars cool, untouched, for 24 hours, then check for a proper seal. You should be able to see that the lids are slightly concave in the center. If you press down in the center and hear a pop, the lid is not secure. If you remove the rings and can easily lift the lid from the jar, the lid is not secure. Any food that hasn't been properly sealed should be refrigerated and used within 3 weeks.

If you live at a high altitude, you must adjust the processing time required for the water bath; add one minute of processing time for each 1,000 feet (305 m) above sea level to account for the fact that water boils at a lower temperature.

Canned foods should be stored below 95°F (35°C); the optimal temperature is between 50°F and 70°F (10°C and 21°C). Properly preserved foods are best when used within 12 months.

Before opening a jar of food that has been preserved, check it for safety. Any jars with cracks, dings in the lids, swelling of lids, or seeping should be discarded immediately. If the lid is not sealed as you open it or there is any mold, growth, or any kind of funky smell, do not taste the food and discard the entire jar.

Acids are very important when canning. Very high-acid fruits (e.g., apples and strawberries) can be canned without added acid, whereas figs and tomatoes require the addition of an acid. If you are unable to use lemon juice or another acid (due to allergies), stick to very high-acid foods, or skip the canning and freeze the food.

Canning equipment essentials

If you plan to preserve foods, you will need a large canning pot with a rack so that the jars don't sit directly on the heat; choose a pot made specifically for this purpose or an 8-quart multipot. Simple tools, including a jar lifter, lid lifter, and wide-mouth funnel, will also make the job a lot easier.

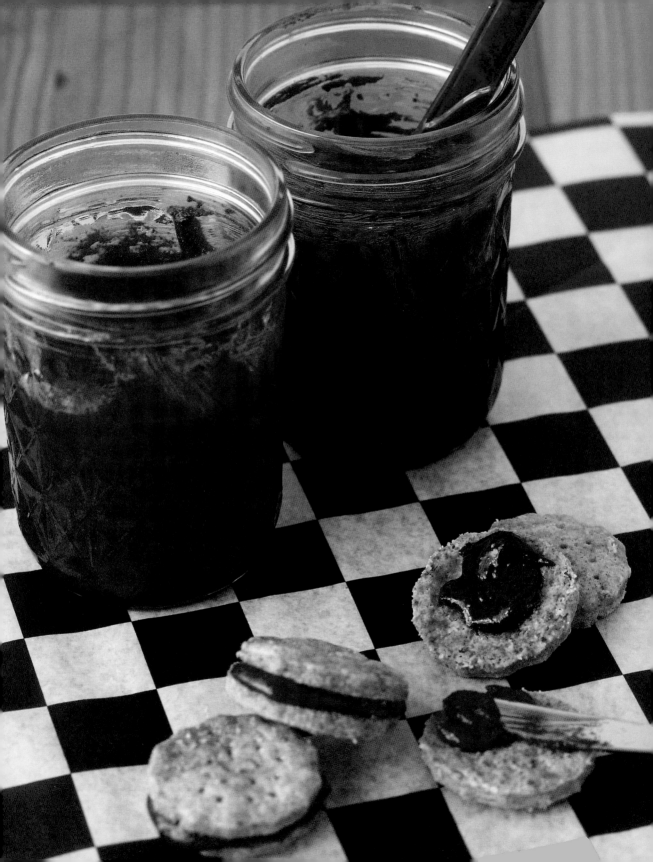

Sunflower Seed Butter

MAKES ABOUT ¾ CUP (175 G)

What to pair with jam? If peanut butter and other nut butters aren't an option, sunflower seed butter is the best alternative I have found. Instead of paying the price for commercially processed sunflower seed butter, try making it at home with this simple recipe. It works best in small batches. Start with roasted sunflower seeds or roast them yourself (see tip below).

1 cup (144 g) shelled, unsalted, roasted sunflower seeds (see below)

¼ teaspoon salt

1½ tablespoons organic cane sugar

1 to 2 tablespoons sunflower oil

1. Place the sunflower seeds and salt in the small bowl of a food processor or blender and process on high for 1½ minutes. Scrape down the sides of the bowl, then let the seeds sit for 15 minutes to release the oils.

2. Add the sugar and process on high for 30 seconds. Scrape down the sides of the bowl and let it sit for 1 minute. Repeat this step three or four times, until the mixture is thick and crumbly.

3. Add the oil ½ tablespoon at a time, blending for a few seconds each time, until the desired consistency is reached. The more oil you add the creamier the butter will be. Store it in an airtight container in the refrigerator for up to 2 months.

HOW TO ROAST SUNFLOWER SEEDS

Preheat the oven to 325°F (165°C). Spread raw, unsalted sunflower seeds on a large baking sheet lined with parchment paper. Roast the seeds for 18 to 20 minutes, until they are fragrant and light golden brown.

Chocolate Sunflower Butter

MAKES ABOUT 1 CUP (285 G)

This combination of sunflower butter and chocolate is reminiscent of Nutella and nothing short of mouthwatering goodness. Spread it on toast for an after-school treat that the whole family can enjoy, or use it to fill Sunflower Butter Cups (page 273) for a double-chocolate treat.

1 cup (144 g) shelled, unsalted, roasted sunflower seeds (see How to Roast Sunflower Seeds on page 77)

¼ teaspoon salt

1½ tablespoons organic cane sugar

½ cup (120 g) chocolate chips

2 to 3 tablespoons sunflower oil

1. Place the sunflower seeds and salt in the small bowl of a food processor or blender and process on high for 1½ minutes. Scrape down the sides of the bowl, then let the seeds sit for 15 minutes to release the oils.

2. Add the sugar and process on high for 30 seconds. Scrape down the sides of the bowl and let it sit for 1 minute. Repeat this step three or four times, until the mixture is thick and oily.

3. Melt the chocolate chips together with 1 tablespoon of oil in a microwave for about 30 seconds, until just melted. Stir to incorporate the oil, then add this to the sunflower mixture. Process on high speed for 30 seconds.

4. Add the remaining oil ½ tablespoon at a time, blending for a few seconds each time, until the desired consistency is reached. The more oil you add the creamier the butter will be.

5. Store it in an airtight container in the refrigerator for up to 2 months. The mixture will harden in the refrigerator. Heat it in the microwave for 10 to 20 seconds to soften.

Apple Butter

I used to think I could find apple butter only at general stores in the quaint towns of New England, but I no longer have to wait for a trip to the mountains to enjoy it. This recipe starts with Applesauce (page 45), builds flavor with sweeteners and spices, and creates spreadable fruit butter by reducing the liquid. The simmering takes time, but your home will smell wonderful, and I think you'll find it's worth the effort.

2¾ cups (660 g) Applesauce (page 45)
¾ cup (180 ml) honey
1 teaspoon Vanilla Extract (page 288)
1 teaspoon ground cinnamon
¼ teaspoon ground cloves
1 tablespoon fresh lemon juice

1. Combine all of the ingredients together in a medium non-reactive saucepan.
2. Bring to a low boil over medium heat, stirring frequently.
3. Turn the heat to low and simmer for approximately 1½ hours, until the mixture is thickened and medium brown in color. Stir every 15 to 20 minutes.
4. If you are canning, start boiling the jars and follow the Steps for Canning on page 74.
5. Continue simmering the apple butter for another 25 to 30 minutes; it is complete when it doesn't fall off of a spoon.
6. If you are canning, fill the jars, leaving ¼ inch (6.5 mm) of headspace, and process them in a water bath for 10 minutes. Otherwise, let the butter cool completely before refrigerating or freezing in airtight containers. Refrigerate for up to 3 weeks or freeze for up to a year; thaw in the refrigerator before using.

TO SUBSTITUTE

Maple syrup may be substituted for honey.

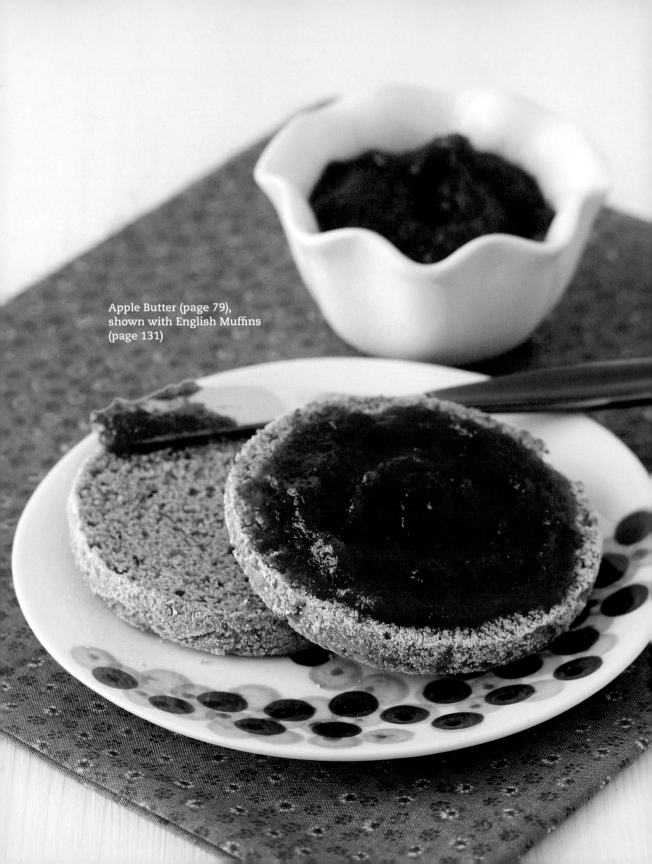

Apple Butter (page 79),
shown with English Muffins
(page 131)

Making Jam

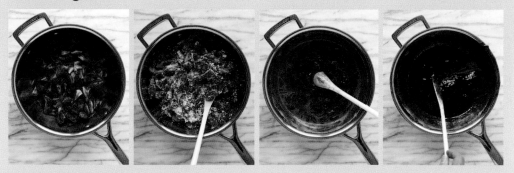

Whether or not you are canning, these are the steps to follow to make jam:

1. Mix the fruit and sugar together in a non-reactive pan and let it sit. The juices from the fruit will be drawn out, the fruit will soften (preparing it for cooking), and the sugar will liquefy. This step can be done up to a day in advance; if you choose to do it ahead, refrigerate the fruit with the sugar in an airtight container.

2. Boil the jam (usually over medium-high heat) until it is thickened. Depending on how much fruit you use, the size of the pan, and how much sugar you use, the timing for this step will vary. Don't be afraid to adjust the timing as needed.

3. Add ingredients, following the recipe. As the jam thickens you will need to stir more frequently. The jam is done when it reaches 220°F (105°C; the temperature at which jam sets), it sheets off of a spoon, or a spoon drawn through the pan leaves a trail or wake for just a second (see rightmost image above). The last method works best if you are using a pan with a large surface area.

If you live at high altitude your jam will set at slightly lower temperatures; subtract 2°F (or 1.1°C) for each 100 feet (or 30 m) you live above sea level.

Freezing is the simplest way of preserving jam; freezing temperatures stop the growth of bacteria. Once the jam is prepared, let it cool, then transfer it to airtight storage containers; leave ½ inch (13 mm) of headspace. Jam can be frozen for up to a year or refrigerated for up to 3 months.

Strawberry Jam

If there is a universal truth about jam, it must be that everyone can agree on strawberry. This is the jam I think of when I think of Sunflower Seed Butter and jam sandwiches, and it's the jam that disappears from my pantry the fastest. June is strawberry season, and that means it's time to pick extra strawberries at the CSA and time to start filling up the pantry shelves with jars of jam.

6 cups (840 g) strawberries, hulled and chopped

2 cups (440 g) organic cane sugar

Two 1-inch (2.5 cm) pieces of vanilla bean, or 1½ teaspoons Vanilla Extract (page 288)

2 tablespoons fresh lemon juice

1. Combine the strawberries and sugar in a medium non-reactive saucepan. Let it sit for an hour until the sugar is partially liquefied.

2. If you are canning, start boiling the jars to be used and follow the Steps for Canning on page 74.

3. Add the vanilla and lemon juice to the strawberries. Boil for about 25 minutes over medium-high heat, stirring occasionally.

4. If using vanilla beans, fish them out and discard them. Boil the jam for another 5 to 10 minutes, until the mixture reaches 220°F (105°C). See Making Jam on page 81 to learn more, including other methods to determine doneness. Skim the foam, if desired.

5. If you are canning, fill the jars, leaving ¼ inch (6.5 mm) of headspace, and process them in a water bath for 10 minutes. Otherwise, let the jam cool completely before refrigerating or freezing in airtight containers. Refrigerate for up to 3 weeks or freeze for up to a year; thaw in the refrigerator.

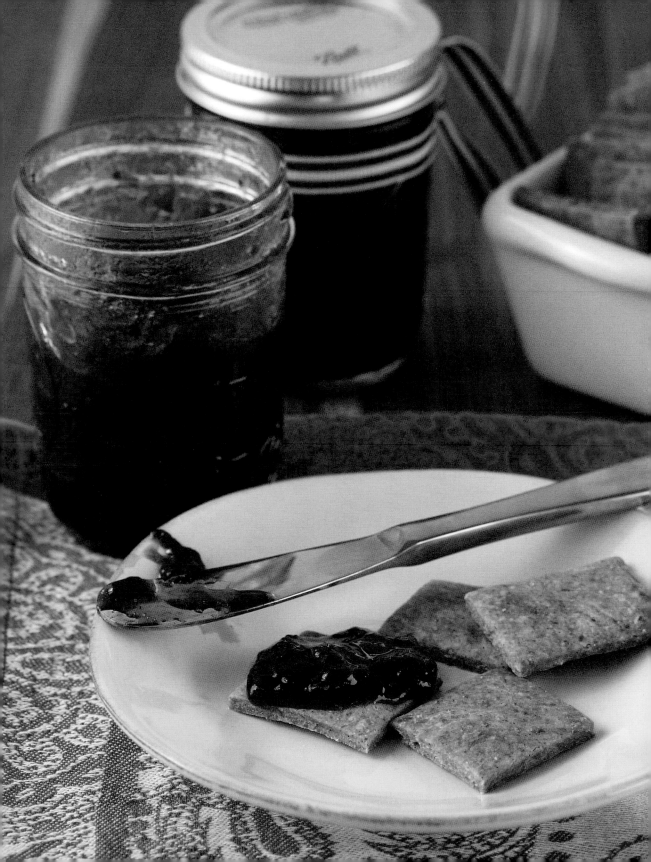

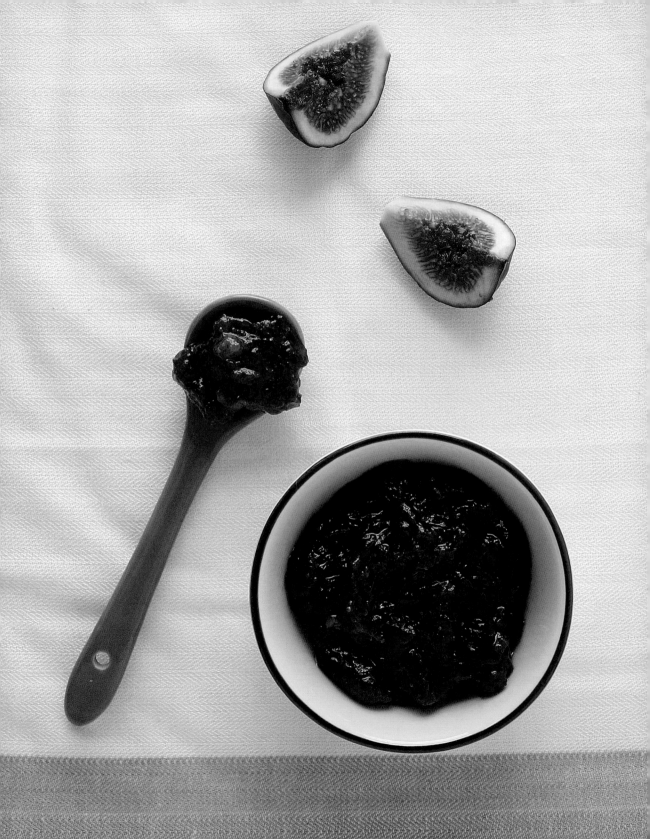

Figgy Pear Jam

MAKES 2½ CUPS (700 G)
Use 2 half-pint (8-ounce/240 ml) and one 4-ounce
(120 ml) jar (or five 4-ounce/120 ml jars) if canning

The sweetness of luscious figs is mellowed a bit by combining it with a pear in this unique jam. The pear also helps to raise the acidity of the figs, but don't leave out the lemon juice if you are canning—it's needed for safe long-term preservation. Use this jam in Fig-Filled Cookies (page 246) or enjoy it on its own.

10 medium figs, stems removed, roughly chopped

1 medium pear, peeled, cored, and diced

1½ cups (330 g) organic cane sugar

2 tablespoons fresh lemon juice

1. Combine the figs, pear, and sugar in a medium non-reactive saucepan. Let it sit for an hour, or until the sugar is partially liquefied.

2. If you are canning, start boiling the jars to be used and follow the Steps for Canning on page 74.

3. Bring the fruit mixture to a boil over medium-high heat, stirring occasionally.

4. After boiling for 10 minutes, use a potato masher to release the seeds and the juice from the fruit. How much you mash depends on how chunky you like your jam.

5. Add the lemon juice and boil for another 3 to 5 minutes, stirring frequently, until the mixture reaches 220°F (105°C). See Making Jam on page 81 to learn more, including other methods to determine doneness.

6. If you are canning, fill the jars, leaving ¼ inch (6.5 mm) of headspace, and process them in a water bath for 10 minutes. Otherwise, let the jam cool completely before refrigerating or freezing in airtight containers. Refrigerate for up to 3 weeks or freeze for up to a year; thaw in the refrigerator.

Honey Blueberry Zest Jam

MAKES 2½ CUPS (700 G)
Use 2 half-pint (8-ounce/240 ml) and one 4-ounce
(120 ml) jar (or five 4-ounce/120 ml jars) if canning

Blueberries are plentiful from early to mid-summer in the Northeast. That's the time to stock up and take advantage of low prices at the grocery store or visit a pick-your-own farm. This chunky jam is kissed with honey and ideal for filling Toaster Tarts (page 129).

4 cups (600 g) blueberries
½ cup (110 g) organic cane sugar
½ cup (120 g) Applesauce (page 45)
½ cup (120 ml) honey
1 tablespoon lemon zest
1 tablespoon fresh lemon juice

1. Crush the blueberries with a potato masher in a medium non-reactive saucepan. Add the sugar and let it sit for 30 minutes.

2. If you are canning, start boiling the jars to be used and follow the Steps for Canning on page 74.

3. Add the applesauce and the honey to the blueberries. Bring the fruit mixture to a boil over medium-high heat, stirring occasionally.

4. After boiling for 10 minutes, add the zest. Lower the heat to medium and boil for 5 minutes longer.

5. Add the lemon juice and boil for another 3 to 5 minutes, stirring frequently, until the mixture reaches 220°F (105°C). See Making Jam on page 81 to learn more, including other methods to determine doneness.

6. If you are canning, fill the jars, leaving ¼ inch (6.5 mm) of headspace, and process them in a water bath for 10 minutes. Otherwise, let the jam cool completely before refrigerating or freezing in airtight containers. Refrigerate for up to 3 weeks or freeze for up to a year; thaw in the refrigerator.

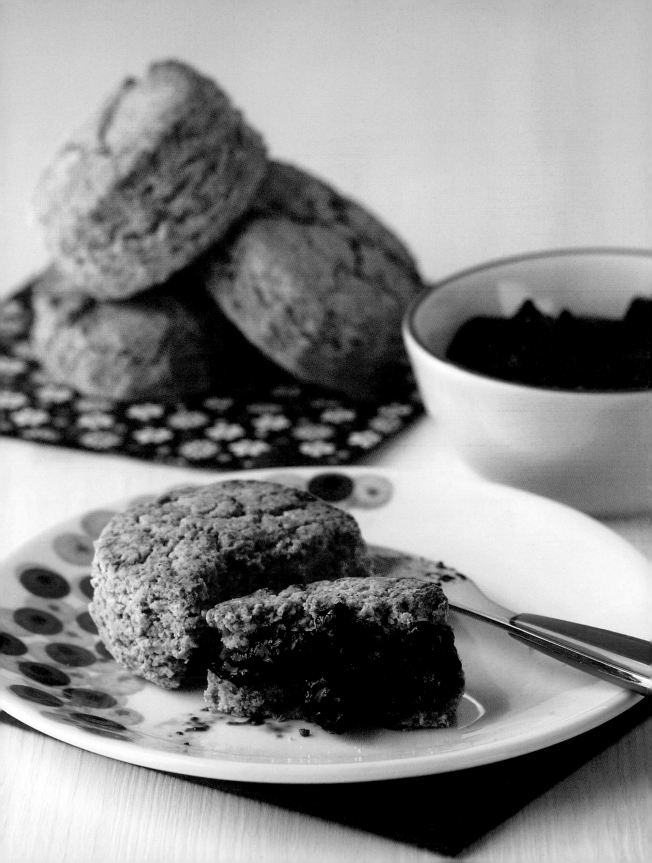

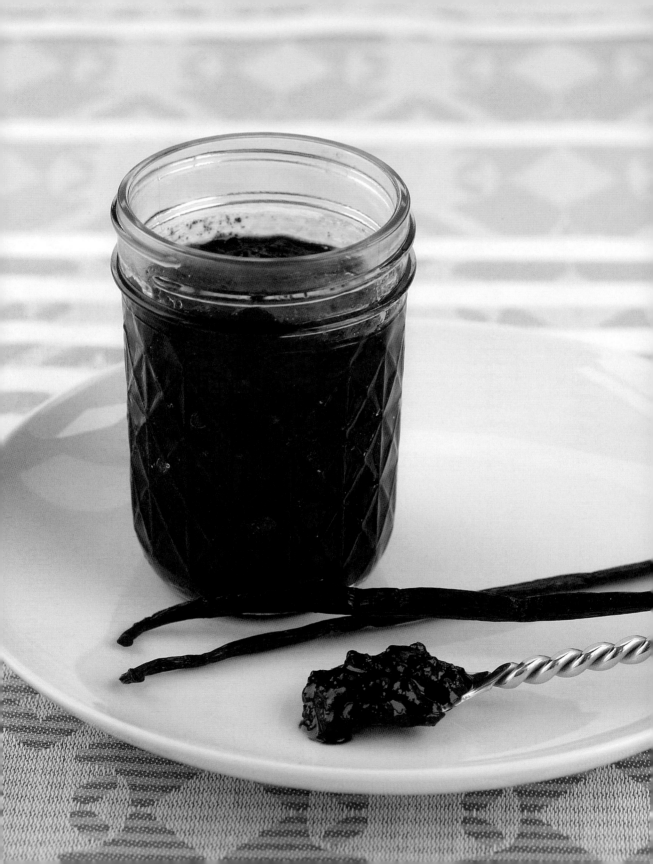

Cherry Vanilla Jam

My husband is a cherry fanatic. Each summer in early June he fills the refrigerator with more cherries than we can eat, inspiring me to create this jam. Sweet or tart, the choice of cherry is yours. Vanilla is the secret ingredient (shhh . . .)!

4 cups (620 g) cherries, pitted and chopped

¾ cup (165 g) sugar

Three 1-inch (2.5 cm) pieces of vanilla bean, or 2 teaspoons Vanilla Extract (page 288)

1 tablespoon fresh lemon juice

1. Combine the cherries and sugar in a medium non-reactive saucepan. Let it sit for an hour, or until the sugar is partially liquefied.

2. If you are canning, start boiling the jars to be used and follow the Steps for Canning on page 74.

3. Add the vanilla to the cherries and boil over medium-high heat for 15 minutes, stirring occasionally.

4. If using vanilla beans, fish them out and discard them. Add the lemon juice. Boil for another 3 to 5 minutes, stirring frequently, until the mixture reaches 220°F (105°C). See Making Jam on page 81 to learn more, including other methods to determine doneness.

5. If you are canning, fill the jars, leaving ¼ inch (6.5 mm) of headspace, and process them in a water bath for 10 minutes. Otherwise, let the jam cool completely before refrigerating or freezing in airtight containers. Refrigerate for up to 3 weeks or freeze for up to a year; thaw in the refrigerator.

7

Condiments *and* Dressings

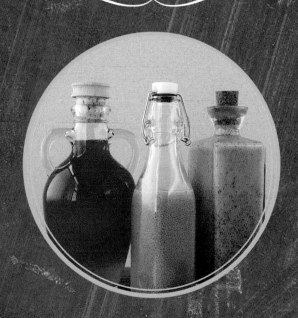

KETCHUP ⌁ MUSTARD ⌁ FLAXSEED MAYONNAISE

CHIPOTLE MAYONNAISE ⌁ SIMPLE VINAIGRETTE ⌁ ITALIAN DRESSING

MOCK CAESAR DRESSING ⌁ DAIRY-FREE RANCH DRESSING

BARBECUE SAUCE ⌁ HONEY MUSTARD SAUCE

The condiment aisle of the grocery store can be a nerve-racking place for those with food allergies. Salad dressings and marinades usually have lengthy, hard-to-read ingredients labels, suspicious ingredients, food colorings, and preservatives, not to mention too much sugar. And the price of allergen-free mayonnaise is often prohibitive—if you can find it at all.

In this chapter you will find flexible recipes that can be tailored to your family's needs. You will still need to walk down the condiment aisle to find single-ingredient items such as oil and vinegar, but you will be able to leave the ketchup, mustard, and salad dressings on the shelf, if you choose to make them at home.

While many of the recipes in this chapter are items that you will want to keep readily available, be aware that shelf lives can vary considerably, depending on the ingredients. For example, a dressing made from oil, vinegar, and sugar will last for up to 6 months; if you add herbs and garlic, the shelf life will be reduced to just a few days. All of the food made from the recipes in this chapter should be refrigerated.

EXPLORING EMULSIONS

Making an emulsion—combining ingredients that do not normally mix—is one of the most fascinating science projects you can do in your kitchen. In this chapter you will find recipes for temporary emulsions, such as salad dressings, as well as more complex permanent emulsions, such as mayonnaise.

To make a temporary emulsion, simply put the ingredients into a jar and shake it vigorously to combine the ingredients. A temporary emulsion can also be created with a whisk and the power of your hand. After sitting for a short time, the ingredients will separate. They can be mixed together again, as needed. We have all seen this dozens of times with salad dressings made from vinegar and oil—two ingredients that don't naturally combine.

A permanent emulsion is much trickier. It requires a specific method and a slow hand. The best example is mayonnaise. Traditional mayonnaise brings together eggs and oil, permanently combining them into a spread. A permanent emulsion requires a stabilizer; in the case of traditional mayonnaise it is the lecithin in the eggs that plays that role. In the case of the mayonnaise recipes I have created for you, Flaxseed Eggs or Chia Seed Eggs (page 42) play that role.

To work properly, a permanent emulsion needs the correct balance of ingredients. Once an emulsion starts to come together, adding more oil will cause it to thicken. Yet, if too much oil is added, the emulsion will "break." This reaction happens quite suddenly; one second you will have a smooth, creamy, spreadable mixture, and the next second it will liquefy. My rule of thumb (when using flaxseed eggs as the stabilizer) is to keep the ratio of flaxseed to oil at 1 to 4 or lower. Each flaxseed egg equals about 3 tablespoons so an emulsion with just one flaxseed egg is prone to break if more than ¾ cup (12 tablespoons/180 ml) of oil is used.

If your emulsion breaks (after it has come together), reduce the amount of oil used next time. In the meantime, instead of throwing away the oil, it may be possible to rescue (or partially rescue) an emulsion that has broken using these steps:

1. Add ½ tablespoon lemon juice and 1 flaxseed egg to a clean working container and pulse them together.
2. Slowly add the broken liquid, starting with a few drops, until the mixture becomes creamy again, then pour the

remaining liquid in a slow trickle. Stop short of adding all the liquid. The result won't be as thick as the original emulsion, but it will be quite suitable as the base for a dip or salad dressing.

Creating an emulsion is challenging, but once you get the hang of it you may feel downright giddy. I suggest trying a couple of practice batches when you're not feeling rushed, using inexpensive oil (e.g., canola oil). Switch to higher-quality oils and experiment with different flavors as you master the technique.

How to Create a Permanent Emulsion

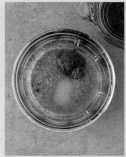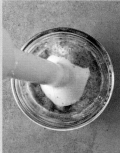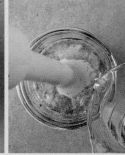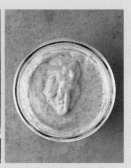

Follow these steps to create a permanent emulsion:

1. Combine the base ingredients (usually everything except the oil), including the protein that will act as a stabilizing agent, in a working glass or the container for your immersion blender. Alternatively, a food processor or blender may be used.

2. Pulse four or five times, until the ingredients are combined.

3. Trickle in the oil, a few drops at a time, while continuously running the blender. After about 1 tablespoon of oil has been added, the mixture will start to become creamy as the fat breaks up (due to the shearing power provided by the blender).

4. Once emulsification has started, the remaining oil can be added a little less slowly. Continue trickling in the oil, moving the stick of the immersion blender up and down (or stopping to stir the ingredients together if using another tool) as needed, until all of the oil is well blended into the mixture.

Ketchup

Fresh tomatoes from your garden or local market can be used here, or you can reduce the time required to make ketchup (and the mess) by using canned crushed tomatoes; make sure you select cans that have just one ingredient—tomatoes. This recipe requires keen attention at the stovetop while the sauce is reducing. Make a big batch of ketchup and preserve some for use throughout the year. Always use peeled tomatoes for safety when preserving, because the skins can harbor bacteria.

1 medium onion, diced

1 medium red bell pepper, diced

2 garlic cloves, minced

6 pounds (2720 g) tomatoes, peeled and seeded (see page 178 to learn how to peel and seed tomatoes), or two 28-ounce (794 g) cans crushed tomatoes

½ cup (120 ml) apple cider vinegar (5 percent acidity)

3 tablespoons organic cane sugar

3 teaspoons salt

½ teaspoon ground black pepper

½ teaspoon ground cinnamon

1. Combine the onion, bell pepper, garlic, and tomatoes in a large pot and bring to a boil over medium heat.

2. Lower the heat to medium-low, cover the pot, and cook until all the vegetables are soft, about 25 minutes.

3. Remove the pot from the heat. Use an immersion blender to puree the vegetables, or transfer the vegetables to a blender and puree.

4. If you are using fresh tomatoes, pass the puree through a fine mesh strainer or food mill to remove any remaining seeds. Discard the seeds. (Skip this step if you are using canned tomatoes.)

5. If you transferred the puree, return it to the pot.

6. Add the vinegar, sugar, and spices and stir all of the ingredients together well. Simmer, uncovered, over medium-low heat for 60 to 90 minutes, until the ketchup is thickened and reduced by half. Stir frequently to avoid making a mess on your stovetop. If you find small bits of vegetables that escaped the blender, fish them out and discard them. If you are canning, start boiling the jars 30 minutes into this step and follow the Steps for Canning on page 74.

7. If you are canning, fill the jars, leaving ½ inch (13 mm) of headspace, and process them in a water bath for 15 minutes. Otherwise, let the ketchup cool, then transfer it to airtight containers; refrigerate for up to 1 month or freeze for up to 6 months. Canned ketchup should be used within a year.

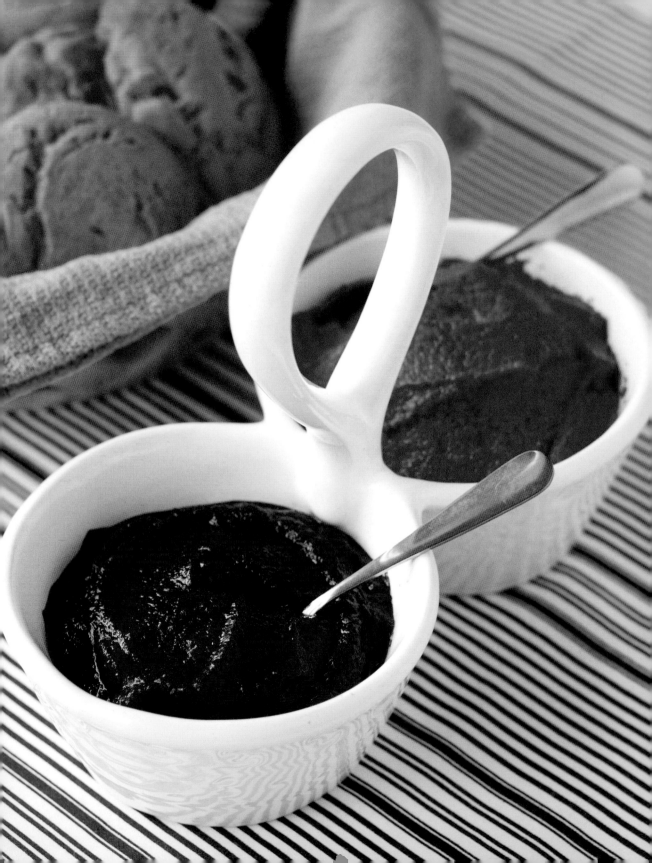

Mustard

Whether you are making Honey Mustard Sauce (page 113) or preparing for a barbecue, this mustard will do the trick. You may find homemade mustard strong at first; the flavor will continue to develop for a few days, and it will mellow over time. Mustard seeds are available in many varieties and colors; feel free to experiment!

¼ cup (46 g) yellow mustard seeds

3 tablespoons brown rice vinegar

½ teaspoon salt

¼ teaspoon ground black pepper

¼ teaspoon turmeric

¼ cup (60 ml) plus up to 3 tablespoons of water

1. Combine all of the dry ingredients with ¼ cup plus 1 tablespoon (75 ml) of water in a working glass or the container for your immersion blender, blender, or food processor. Let it sit in the refrigerator, covered, for at least 12 hours or up to 3 days.

2. After soaking, pulse to combine the ingredients, then puree. You can control how smooth or chunky your mustard is. Add up to 2 more tablespoons of water and continue to puree until the desired consistency is reached.

3. Cover and refrigerate for up to 3 months.

VARIATION

To make Dijon Mustard, substitute white wine vinegar and white wine for the brown rice vinegar and water, respectively.

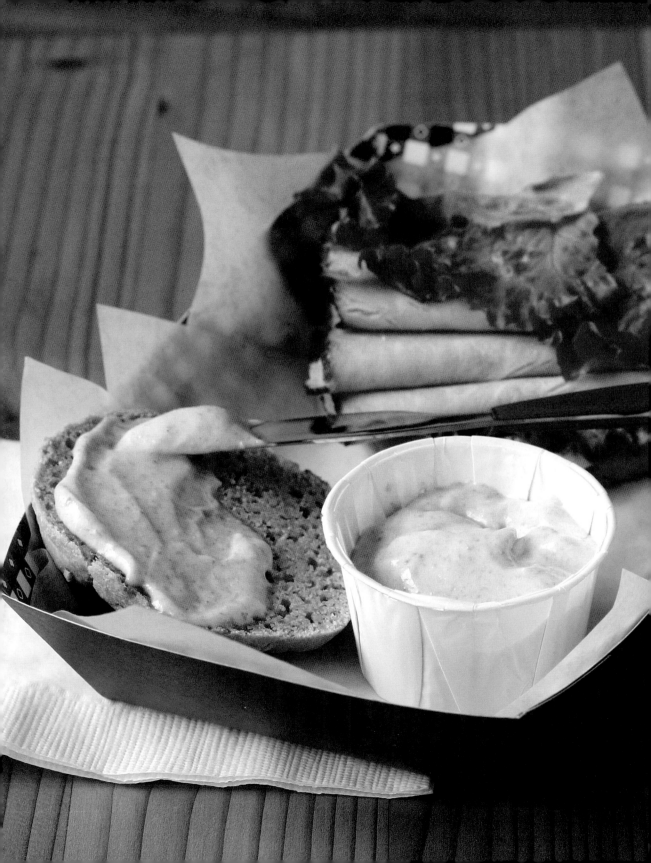

Flaxseed Mayonnaise

Because this mayonnaise starts with flaxseeds rather than eggs, it has the benefit of being both healthier and tastier than traditional mayonnaise. Even if you aren't allergic to eggs, this might just be the best sandwich topping you have ever tried!

Use measuring cups with a spout to measure the oil; this will allow you to pour the oil directly into the container for your blender when making mayonnaise.

2 Flaxseed Eggs (page 42)

½ teaspoon salt

1 teaspoon Mustard (page 97), or ¼ teaspoon ground mustard seed

1 tablespoon fresh lemon juice

½ cup (120 ml) organic canola oil

¼ cup (60 ml) light olive oil

1. Combine the flaxseed eggs, salt, mustard, and lemon juice in a working glass or the container for your immersion blender, blender, or food processor. Pulse four or five times to combine the ingredients.

2. With the blender running continuously, pour a few drops of canola oil into the container. The slower you pour, the better. The mixture will start to become creamy as emulsification occurs.

3. Continue blending and adding oil in a slow trickle until all of the oil is incorporated; add all of the canola oil first and then the olive oil. If the oil starts to pool on top of the mixture, slide your immersion blender up and down ½ inch, or stop pouring until the oil combines. See How to Create a Permanent Emulsion on page 94.

4. Cover and refrigerate for up to 1 week. The mixture will set further as it chills.

TO SUBSTITUTE

A single oil or any combination of oils (up to ¾ cup/180 ml total) can be used to make this mayonnaise, with the exception of coconut oil or palm fruit oil (which behave differently). Use less oil for a thinner spread.

VARIATION

Make Chia Seed Mayonnaise by substituting 2 Chia Seed Eggs (page 42) for the Flaxseed Eggs.

Chipotle Mayonnaise

That delicious, creamy, salmon-colored mayonnaise or dip served at chain restaurants doesn't have to be off-limits at home. This tangy mayonnaise works as a sandwich spread, and it's also the perfect complement to Onion Rings (page 163).

2 Flaxseed Eggs (page 42)

1 teaspoon salt

1 teaspoon ground chipotle chile powder

2 garlic cloves, minced

2 tablespoons fresh lime juice

½ cup (120 ml) grapeseed oil

¼ cup (60 ml) organic canola oil

1. Combine the flaxseed eggs, salt, chipotle powder, garlic, and lime juice in a working glass or the container for your immersion blender, blender, or food processor. Pulse four or five times to combine the ingredients.

2. Combine the oils in a single measuring cup with a spout.

3. With the blender running continuously, pour a few drops of oil into the container.

The slower you pour, the better. The mixture will start to become creamy as emulsification occurs.

4. Continue blending and adding oil in a slow trickle until all of the oil is incorporated. If the oil starts to pool on top of the mixture, slide your immersion blender up and down ½ inch or stop pouring until the oil combines. See How to Create a Permanent Emulsion on page 94.

5. Cover and refrigerate for up to 1 week. The mixture will set further as it chills.

TO SUBSTITUTE

A single oil or any combination of oils (up to ¾ cup/180 ml total) can be used to make this mayonnaise, with the exception of coconut oil or palm fruit oil (which behave differently).

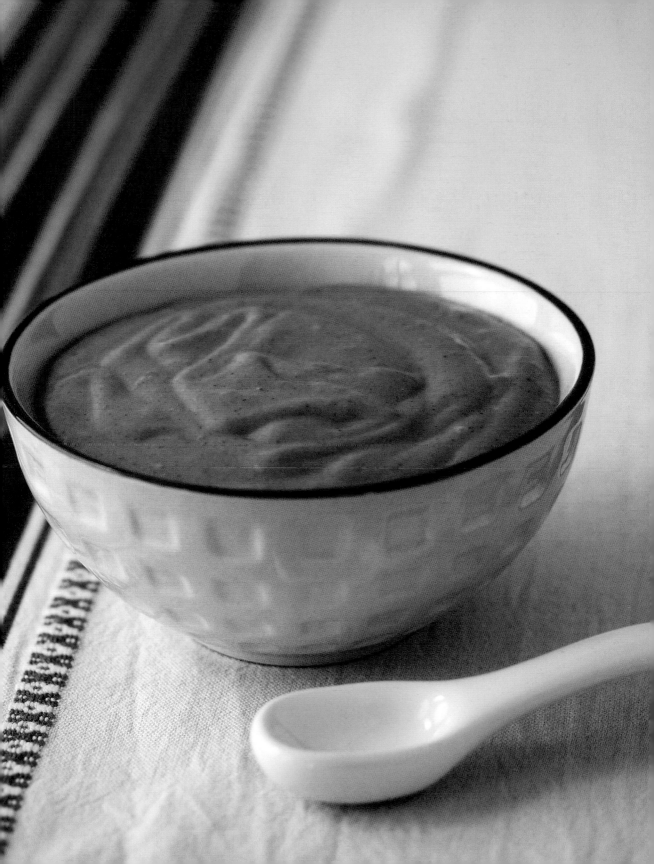

Simple Vinaigrette

Vinaigrette is the simplest of the salad dressings, and a basic from which you can create a variety of flavors. The standard formula for vinaigrette is 3 parts oil to 1 part vinegar (or acid), but this is a rule that's meant to be broken. Feel free to vary the ratios (as I have done here), to substitute different oils or acids, and to modify the type and amount of sweetener used (or leave it out completely).

Over time you will learn to make salad dressing without a measuring cup, simply by eyeballing the amounts as you pour them into the jar to shake.

¾ cup (180 ml) light olive oil
½ cup (120 ml) brown rice vinegar
2 tablespoons agave nectar
½ teaspoon salt

1. Combine all of the ingredients in a jar, cover, and shake them together. Alternatively, a whisk, a blender, food processor, or immersion blender can be used to combine the ingredients.

2. Refrigerate for up to 6 months. Shake to recombine the ingredients before each use.

VARIATION

To make Raspberry Vinaigrette, add 4 to 5 crushed raspberries (fresh or frozen, including the juice) to the dressing. Cover and shake well. Refrigerate for up to 5 days.

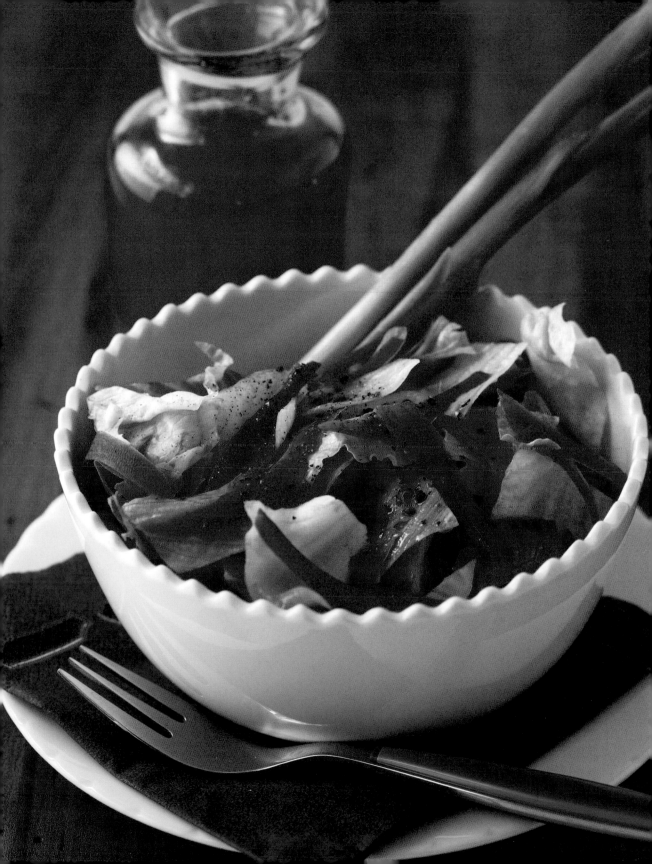

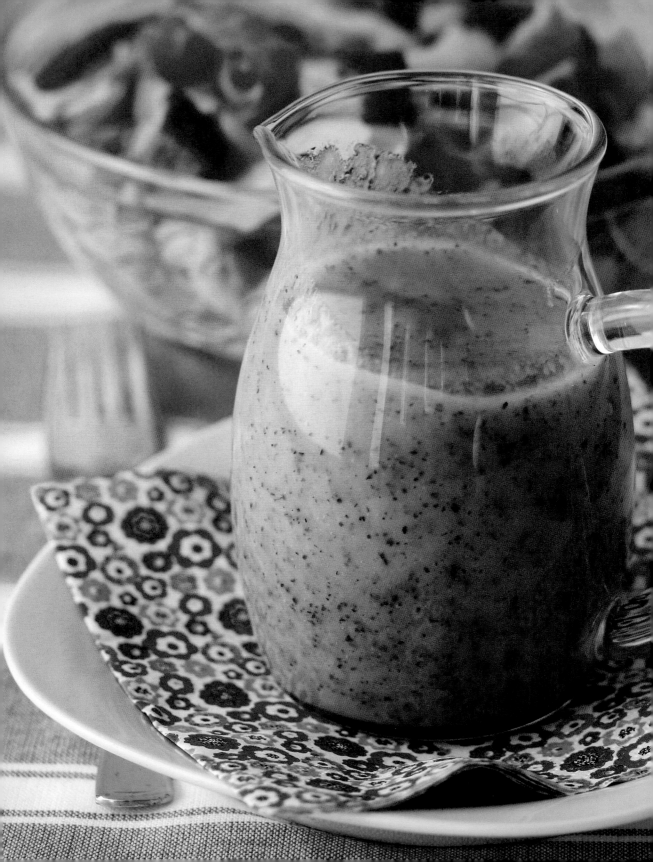

Italian Dressing

It's the garlic and herbs that make Italian dressing special. Prepare it ahead so that you have time to let the herbs infuse into the dressing before tossing it with the salad.

¼ cup plus 1 tablespoon (75 ml) white wine vinegar

1 garlic clove, minced

½ teaspoon dried oregano

½ tablespoon chopped fresh parsley

½ tablespoon chopped fresh basil

½ teaspoon salt

¼ teaspoon ground black pepper

1¼ cups (300) light olive oil

1. Combine all of the ingredients except the oil in a working glass or the container for your immersion blender, blender, or food processor. Pulse four or five times until the ingredients are combined.

2. Slowly add the oil and process until creamy. A temporary emulsion will form. Refrigerate for up to 5 days in a covered jar or working glass.

Mock Caesar Dressing

This temporary emulsion leaves out the anchovies and the egg, yet it tastes remarkably similar to traditional Caesar dressing. The hemp seeds give the dressing some texture and a mild cheesy taste.

1 garlic clove, minced

¼ teaspoon ground black pepper

¼ teaspoon salt

1½ tablespoons fresh lemon juice

1 teaspoon Mustard (page 97), or ¼ teaspoon ground mustard seed

1 tablespoon Flaxseed Mayonnaise (page 99)

2 tablespoons shelled hemp seeds

⅔ cup (160 ml) light olive oil

1. Combine all of the ingredients except the oil in the container for an immersion blender, blender, or food processor. Pulse four or five times until the ingredients are combined.

2. Slowly add the oil and process until creamy. A temporary emulsion will form. Refrigerate for up to 5 days in a covered jar or working glass.

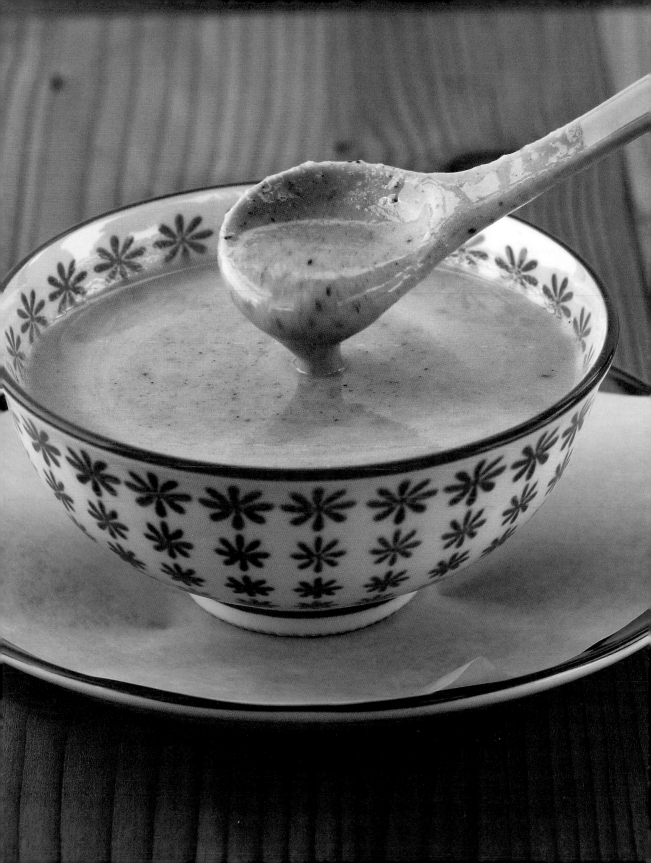

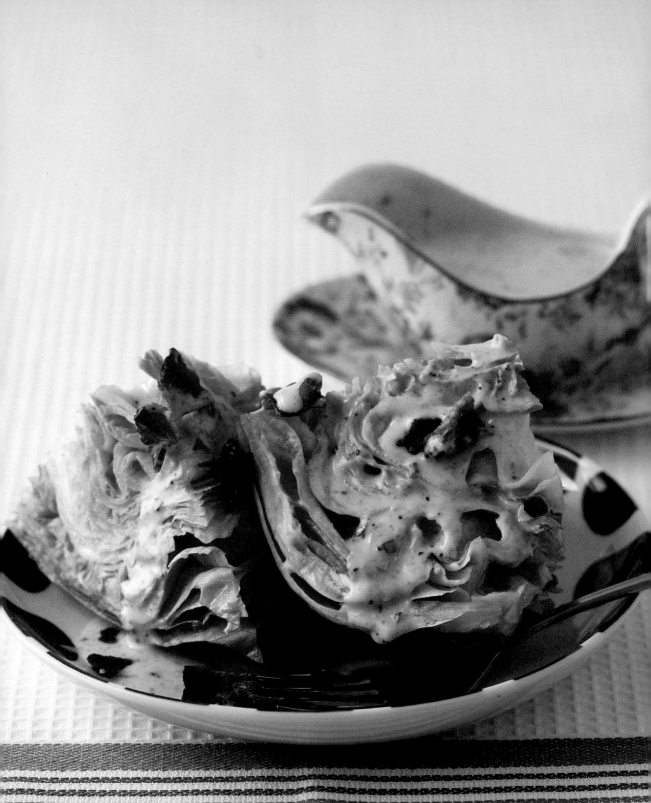

Dairy-Free Ranch Dressing

MAKES ¾ CUP (180 ML)

I wasn't surprised to learn that ranch dressing is the most popular salad dressing in North America. Whether it's to top a wedge salad or to serve as a dip with fresh vegetables, ranch is the dressing you will turn to time after time. This dairy-free recipe leverages Flaxseed Mayonnaise to make a creamy emulsion.

½ cup (120 ml) Flaxseed Mayonnaise (page 99)

2 tablespoons light olive oil

2 tablespoons fresh lemon juice

½ teaspoon ground black pepper

½ teaspoon finely grated onion

½ teaspoon finely grated garlic

1 teaspoon minced chives

1. Whisk together the mayonnaise, oil, and lemon juice in a medium bowl.

2. Add the pepper, onion, garlic, and chives and whisk them in. Refrigerate for up to 5 days in a covered jar or working glass.

Barbecue Sauce

Start with homemade Ketchup (page 95), add spices, simmer for a bit, and you will have barbecue sauce that rivals anything you might find off the shelf. I chose Sucanat (see page 8) for this recipe because it is whole sugar, retaining all of its natural molasses; if you need a substitute, use brown sugar.

2 cups (420 g) Ketchup (page 95)
¼ cup (42 g) Sucanat
¼ cup (60 ml) apple cider vinegar
½ teaspoon ground black pepper
½ teaspoon ground chipotle chile powder
2 garlic cloves, finely grated

1. Combine all of the ingredients in a medium non-reactive saucepan. Bring to a boil over medium heat.

2. Turn the heat to low and simmer for 20 to 25 minutes, stirring occasionally, until slightly thickened.

3. Use the sauce immediately, or allow it to cool to room temperature and then refrigerate it in an airtight container for up to 1 week.

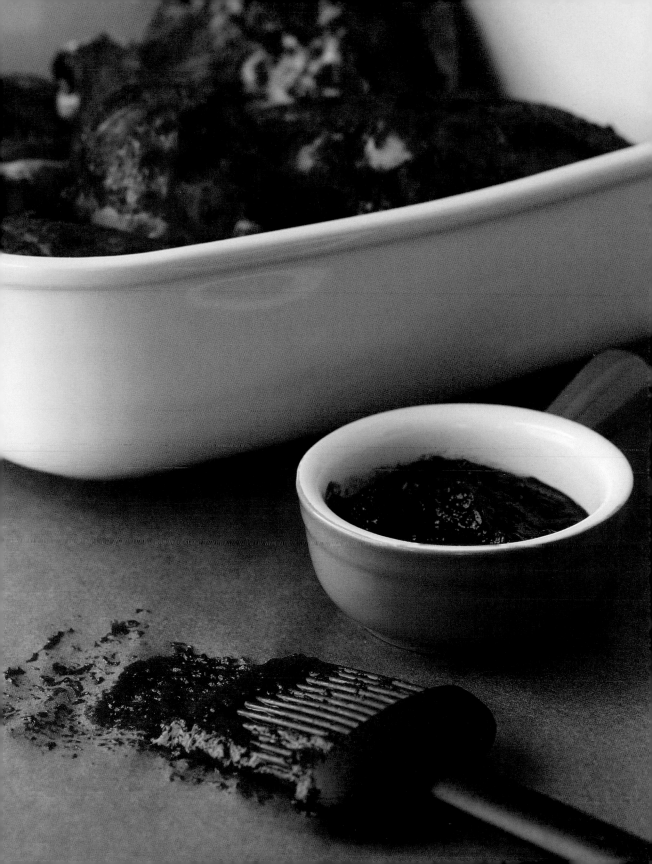

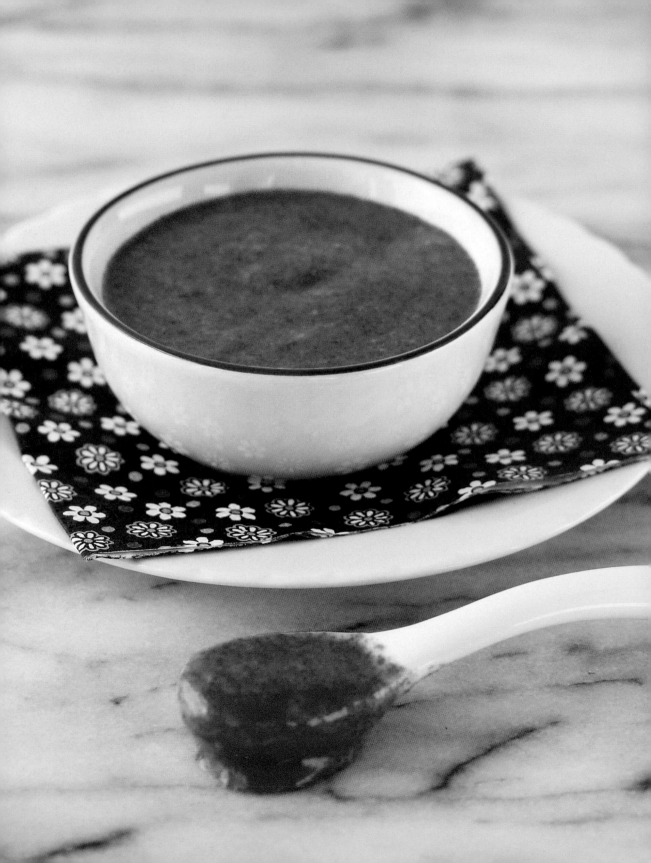

Honey Mustard Sauce

This easy sauce can be used as a dipping sauce for Soft-Baked Pretzel Bites (page 206) or Chicken Tenders (page 191) and can also be used to make a salad dressing or marinade (see variation). If you have a safe off-the-shelf mustard in your pantry, you can use it in place of the homemade version.

¼ cup (60 ml) honey
¼ cup (54 g) Mustard (page 97)
¼ cup (60 ml) sunflower oil
⅛ teaspoon ground black pepper

1. Combine the honey and mustard in a working glass or the container for your immersion blender, blender, or food processor. Pulse until the ingredients are combined.
2. Slowly add the oil and process until creamy. An emulsion will form. (See How to Create a Permanent Emulsion on page 94.)
3. Add pepper to taste. Cover and refrigerate for up to 3 months.

VARIATION

Make Honey Mustard Dressing/Marinade by whisking together ¼ cup (60 ml) Honey Mustard Sauce with ¾ cup (180 ml) light olive oil and ¼ cup (60 ml) brown rice vinegar.

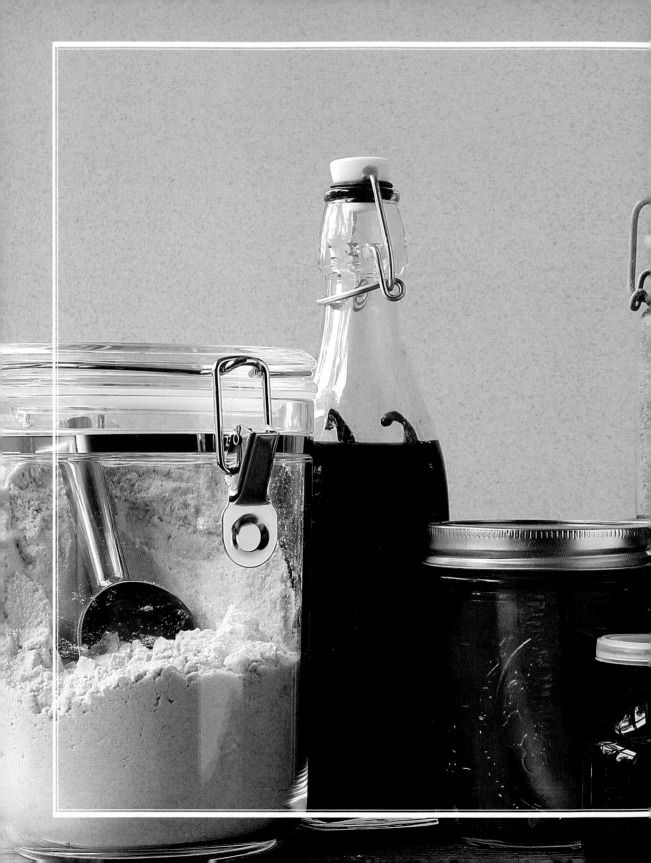

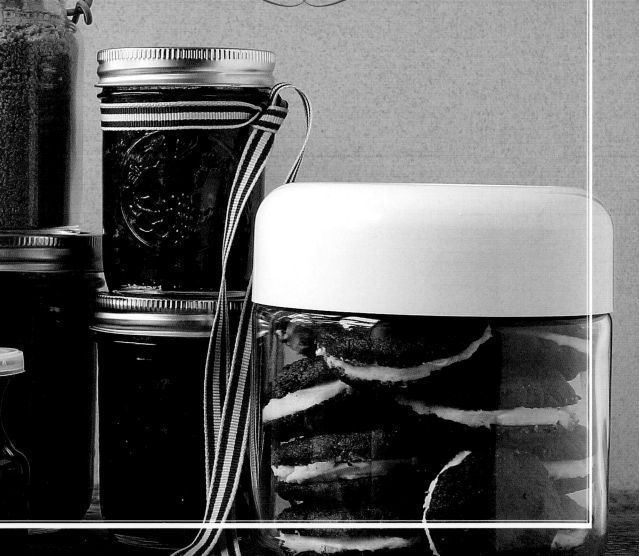

PART

2

MEALS

8.

Breakfast

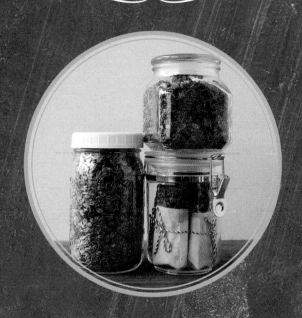

PANCAKES ∂ RASPBERRY MAPLE SYRUP ∂ POWDERED DOUGHNUT HOLES

APPLE OATMEAL SCONES ∂ CHOCOLATE CHIP COOKIE DOUGH MUFFINS

TOASTER TARTS ∂ ENGLISH MUFFINS ∂ CRANBERRY MAPLE GRANOLA

HONEY BLUEBERRY GRANOLA ∂ CHOCOLATE RAISIN

GRANOLA BARS ∂ POLENTA (GRITS)

Breakfast can be a challenge for many with food allergies. Cereals, muffins, and pancakes are traditionally made with wheat and dairy, and eggs are off the table. Whether you are craving English Muffins (page 131), Toaster Tarts (page 129), or nut-free granola, you will find recipes for them here. Hold on to your hats, because breakfast is about to become your favorite meal—again!

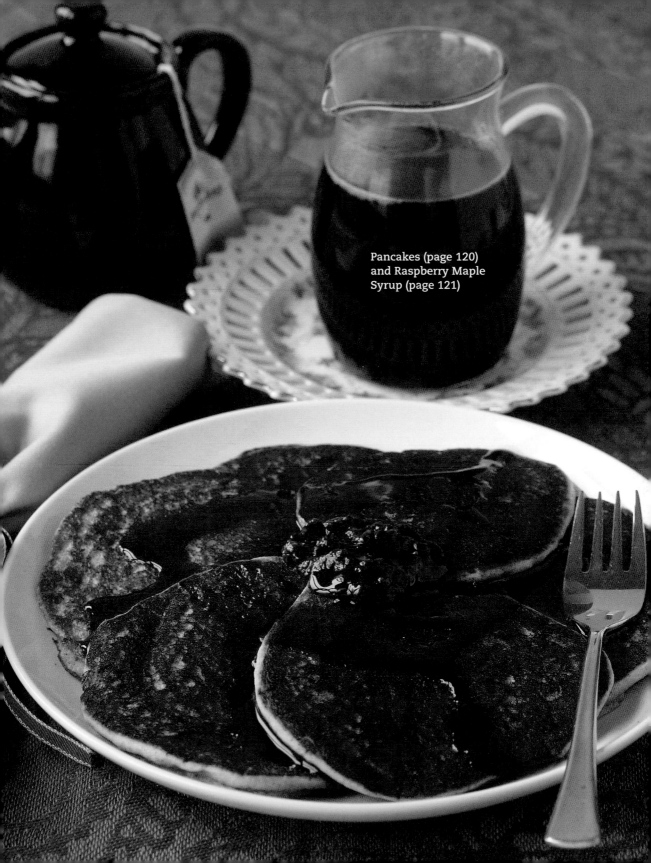

Pancakes (page 120)
and Raspberry Maple
Syrup (page 121)

Pancakes

My family's choice of breakfast on special occasions, holidays, and the occasional lazy Sunday is pancakes. Serve them plain with pure maple syrup, add your favorite in-season fruit to the batter, or top them with Raspberry Maple Syrup (opposite page). Freeze them in pairs in airtight bags and you have the solution for a quick midweek breakfast.

3 tablespoons grapeseed oil plus more for pan

1 Flaxseed Egg (page 42)

1¾ to 2 cups (420 to 480 ml) Hemp Milk (page 31) or non-dairy milk of choice

1 teaspoon Vanilla Extract (page 288)

300 grams (about 2¼ cups) Pancake and Baking Mix (page 24)

1. Whisk together 3 tablespoons of oil, flaxseed egg, 1¾ cups (420 ml) of milk, and vanilla.

2. Whisk in the Pancake and Baking Mix. Add up to ¼ cup (60 ml) more milk until the desired consistency is reached.

3. Heat a small amount of oil in a skillet over medium-high heat.

4. Spoon the pancake batter, in portions, into the skillet. Flip the pancakes when you can see small holes forming in the tops of the pancakes. Cook for 1 to 2 minutes longer, until lightly browned.

5. Repeat step 4 with additional batter. Add more oil to the pan as needed to avoid sticking.

TO FREEZE

Cooked pancakes can be frozen in airtight containers for up to 3 months. Thaw in the refrigerator and reheat in the oven or toaster oven at 325°F (165°C) for 10 minutes.

TO SUBSTITUTE

If you need to replace the flaxseed egg in pancakes, use Ener-G Egg Replacer (see page 41).

A NOTE ABOUT WAFFLES

I don't recommend making egg-free waffles, as the batter will stick mercilessly to most waffle irons.

Raspberry Maple Syrup

MAKES 1 CUP (240 ML)

Top your pancakes with this fresh fruit syrup and everyone will think you made a trip to the gourmet shop. This recipe can be made with any combination of soft berries. If you choose frozen berries, thaw them first; use all of the liquid, and reduce the water to compensate.

1 cup (124 g) raspberries
¼ cup (55 g) organic cane sugar
½ tablespoon fresh lemon juice
¼ cup (60 ml) water
¾ cup (180 ml) pure maple syrup

1. Combine the berries, sugar, lemon juice, and water in a small non-reactive saucepan over medium-low heat. Stir occasionally until the sugar is melted. Heat for 10 minutes more, stirring frequently.

2. Place a fine mesh strainer over a bowl. Use the strainer to separate the fruit and seeds from the juice. Save the fruit to top the pancakes, or refrigerate it and use it as jam.

3. Return the strained liquid to the saucepan. Add the maple syrup and heat over low heat until the pancakes are ready to serve. Refrigerate syrup for up to 2 weeks.

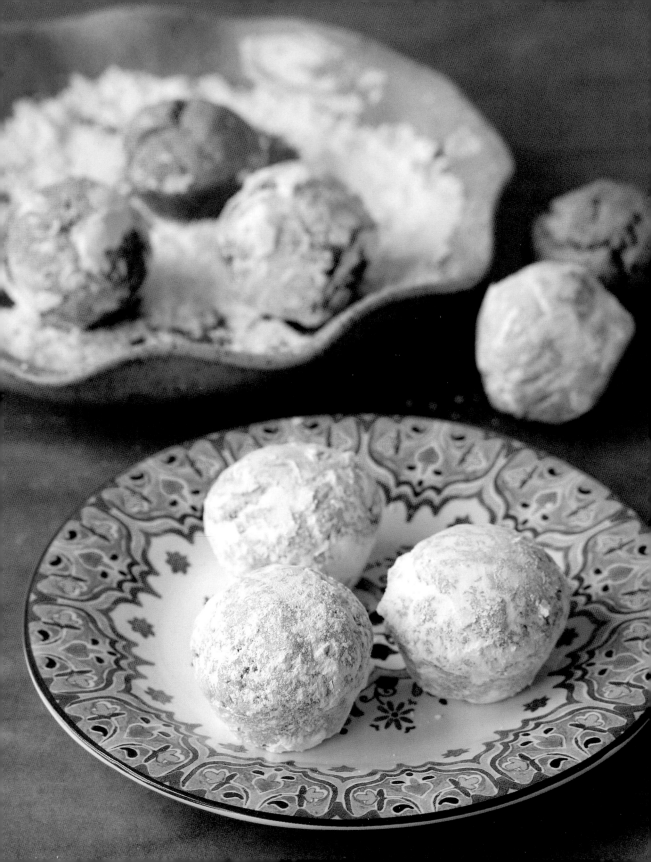

Powdered Doughnut Holes

||||||||||||||||||||||||||||||||||||||||||||||||||||||||||||||||||||||||||||||||||||||||||||||||||||||||||||||||||||||||||||||||||||||||||||

This is the solution for an early-morning status meeting or an allergen-free classroom treat. These muffins have that classic old-fashioned doughnut taste and are easily made in less than 30 minutes using a mini-muffin pan or doughnut hole pan.

288 grams (about 2¼ cups) Basic Flour Blend (page 23)

½ teaspoon xanthan gum

3 teaspoons baking powder

½ teaspoon salt

4 tablespoons shortening (see page 7), softened

½ cup (110 g) organic cane sugar

1 Flaxseed Egg (page 42)

¼ cup (60 ml) Hemp Milk (page 31) or non-dairy milk of choice

½ cup (120 g) Applesauce (page 45)

2 tablespoons grapeseed oil

1 teaspoon Vanilla Extract (page 288)

½ cup (72 g) Powdered Sugar (page 286)

1. Preheat the oven to 350°F (180°C). Grease the cups of a mini-muffin pan or dough-nut hole pan.

2. Combine the flour, xanthan gum, baking powder, and salt in a medium bowl.

3. In a separate large bowl, cream together the shortening and sugar using a mixer on medium speed for 5 minutes. Scrape down the sides of the mixing bowl, as needed.

4. Add the flaxseed egg and blend on medium speed for 1 minute. Add the milk, applesauce, oil, and vanilla, and blend for another minute.

5. Add the dry ingredients and mix on medium speed for 2 to 3 minutes, until well blended. The batter will be thick with some graininess.

6. Use a #40 cookie scoop or spoon to form balls of dough in tablespoon-sized por-tions. Dampen your hands with warm water and gently pass the dough from hand to hand until the ball is smooth. Place each ball of dough into the prepared pan. Dip the cookie scoop or spoon into warm water periodically, if the dough starts to stick.

7. Bake for 14 to 16 minutes, until a tooth-pick inserted comes out clean.

8. Let the doughnut holes cool for 5 minutes in the pan, then transfer them to a cool-ing rack.

9. Just prior to serving, roll the doughnut holes in the powdered sugar to coat them on all sides or sprinkle the powdered sugar on just the tops. Store (without the powdered sugar topping) in an airtight container at room temperature for 2 to 3 days.

VARIATION

To make Cinnamon Sugar Doughnut Holes, sprinkle the tops of the doughnut holes with 3 tablespoons Cinnamon Sugar (page 286) prior to baking. Omit the powdered sugar.

TO FREEZE

Freeze unpowdered doughnut holes for up to 6 months in an airtight container. Thaw at room temperature. Reheat at 325°F (165°C) for 7 min-utes and then add powdered sugar, if desired.

Apple Oatmeal Scones

These hearty scones make a delicious and seasonal breakfast in the fall, when apples are plentiful. Serve them as an alternative to cereal, granola, or hot oatmeal. Take the apple flavor over the top by spreading them with Apple Butter (page 79).

¾ cup (75 g) Granny Smith apple, peeled, cored, and cut into ¼-inch (6.5 mm) cubes

1 tablespoon fresh lemon juice

192 grams (about 1½ cups) Basic Flour Blend (page 23)

56 grams (about ½ cup) gluten-free oat flour

½ teaspoon xanthan gum

2 teaspoons baking powder

1 teaspoon baking soda

½ teaspoon salt

¼ cup (60 ml) grapeseed oil

½ cup (120 g) Applesauce (page 45)

¼ cup (60 ml) honey

¼ cup (60 ml) apple juice

1 tablespoon gluten-free old-fashioned rolled oats

1 tablespoon Cinnamon Sugar (page 286)

1. Preheat the oven to 350°F (180°C). Grease the cups of a scone pan or line a large baking sheet with parchment paper.

2. Toss the apples with the lemon juice in a small bowl and set them aside.

3. Combine the flours, xanthan gum, baking powder, baking soda, and salt in a medium bowl.

4. In a separate large bowl, combine the oil, applesauce, honey, and juice using a mixer on medium speed for 1 minute.

5. Add the dry ingredients and mix for about 2 minutes on medium-low, until a thick batter forms. Stir in the apples by hand.

6. If you are using a scone pan, spoon the batter evenly into the cups of the pan. Otherwise, sprinkle a few drops of water on a smooth prep surface and scoop the dough on top. Use wet fingers to smooth the dough into a round disk. Use a bench knife (see tool tip on page 132) or sharp knife to cut the disk into eight wedges (as you would cut pizza slices) and transfer them to the prepared baking sheet, evenly spaced.

7. Toss the oats with the cinnamon sugar and sprinkle them on top of the scones.

8. Bake for 19 to 21 minutes, until a toothpick inserted comes out clean. Store the scones in an airtight container at room temperature for 2 to 3 days.

TO FREEZE

Freeze scones in an airtight container for up to 6 months. Thaw at room temperature; reheat at 325°F (165°C) for 7 minutes.

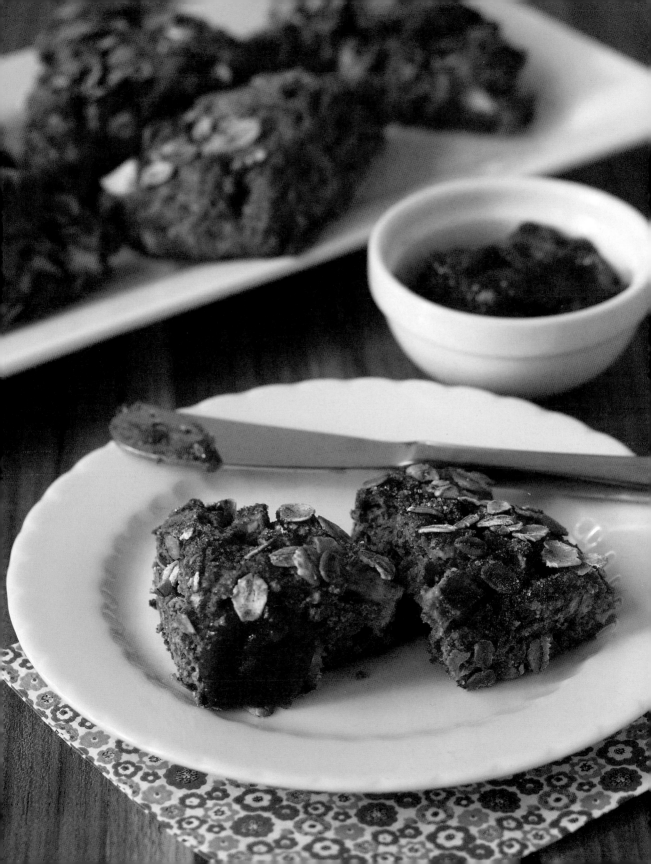

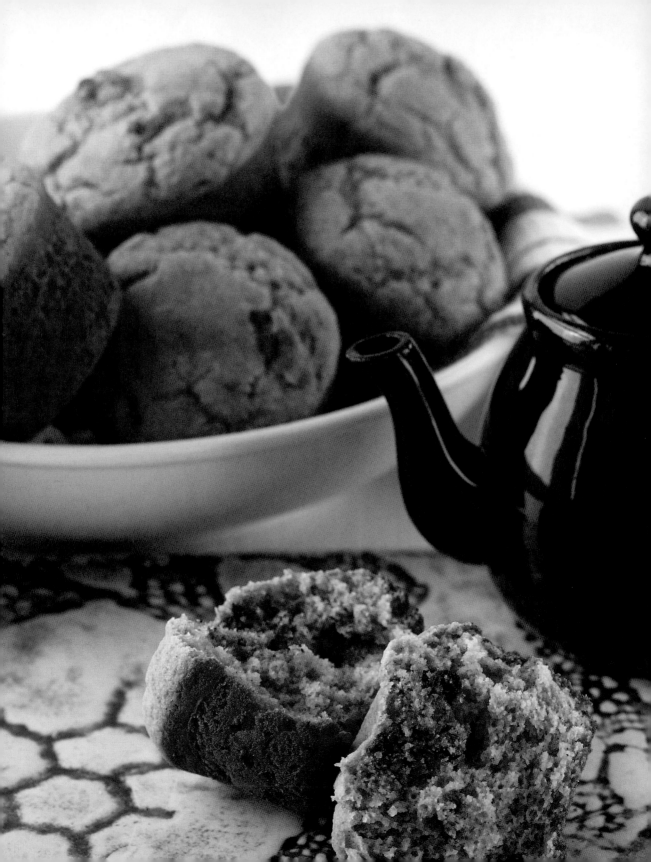

Chocolate Chip Cookie Dough Muffins

MAKES 12 MUFFINS

*B*ite into one of these muffins and you will find a nice surprise—bits of chocolate chip cookies baked right in! Make Chocolate Chip Cookies (page 238) today, save some dough, and you'll be ready to make these muffins for breakfast tomorrow morning. Use another refrigerated cookie dough (e.g., the chocolate dough used to make Chocolate Sandwich Cookies, page 241) to create your own version of cookie dough muffins.

256 grams (about 2 cups) Basic Flour Blend (page 23)

½ teaspoon xanthan gum

3 teaspoons baking powder

1 teaspoon salt

½ cup (110 g) organic cane sugar

½ cup (120 g) Applesauce (page 45)

¼ cup (60 ml) grapeseed oil

1 cup (240 ml) Hemp Milk (page 31) or non-dairy milk of choice

1 teaspoon Vanilla Extract (page 288)

¼ batch (½ roll) of refrigerated Chocolate Chip Cookie dough (page 238)

1. Preheat the oven to 350°F (180°C). Grease the cups of a muffin pan.
2. Combine the flour, xanthan gum, baking powder, salt, and sugar in a medium bowl.
3. In a separate large bowl, combine the applesauce, oil, milk, and vanilla using a mixer on medium speed for 1 minute.
4. Add the dry ingredients and mix on medium speed until the batter is smooth, about 2 minutes.
5. Slice the cookie dough into ¼-inch (6.5 mm) slices, then divide each slice into four pieces. Use your fingers to tightly pack each piece into a ball. Stir the cookie dough pieces into the batter, by hand.
6. Spoon the batter into the cups of the prepared muffin pan. Bake for 21 to 22 minutes, until a toothpick inserted comes out clean.
7. Let the muffins cool for 5 minutes in the muffin pan, then transfer them to a cooling rack. Store in an airtight container at room temperature for 2 to 3 days.

TO FREEZE

Muffins that won't be eaten within 2 to 3 days can be frozen in an airtight container for up to 6 months. Thaw and reheat at 325°F (165°C) for 7 minutes.

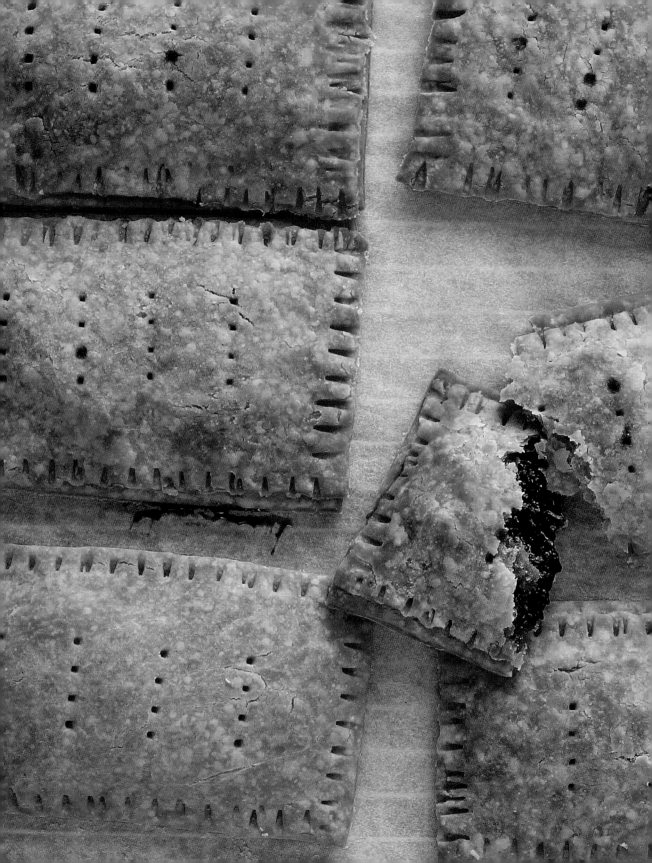

Toaster Tarts

||||||||||||||||||||||||||||||||||||||||||||||||||||||||||||||||||||||||||||||||||||||||||||||||||||||||||||||||||||||||||||||||||||||||||

It's a breakfast classic. Whether you like yours frosted or plain, this food-allergy-friendly version makes a yummy breakfast for busy days. Make Toaster Tarts on the weekend and freeze them; thaw them the night before and you'll just need to heat and go in the morning. Choose your favorite jam to fill these tarts. Frost them only when you are ready to serve.

260 grams (about 2 cups) Pastry Flour Blend (page 24)

½ teaspoon xanthan gum

2 tablespoons organic cane sugar

½ teaspoon salt

8 tablespoons shortening (see page 7), cold

2 tablespoons Applesauce (page 45)

½ teaspoon Vanilla Extract (page 288)

¼ cup (60 ml) plus 2 tablespoons cold water

½ cup (115 to 125 g) Honey Blueberry Zest Jam (page 86), Cherry Vanilla Jam (page 89), or jam of choice

1. Combine the flour, xanthan gum, sugar, and salt in a large mixing bowl.

2. Cut the shortening into tablespoon-sized pieces and lay them on top of the flour. Use a pastry cutter, a pastry fork, or your hands to work the shortening into the flour. Continue working for 3 to 4 minutes, until a crumbly mixture forms.

3. Add the applesauce, vanilla, and ¼ cup (60 ml) water. Work the liquids into the dough using the pastry cutter. Add up to 2 more tablespoons of cold water as needed, ½ tablespoon at a time, until the dough is smooth and pliable.

4. Separate the dough into two sections and form each section into a disk about ½ inch (13 mm) thick. Wrap them tightly in plastic and refrigerate for at least an hour. Pastry dough can be refrigerated for up to 2 weeks.

5. When you are ready to make the tarts, preheat the oven to 350°F (180°C). Line a large baking sheet with parchment paper.

6. Roll out the first section of dough between two sheets of parchment paper. Use additional flour, if needed, to avoid sticking.

7. Cut eight 2½ by 4-inch (6.5 by 10 cm) rectangular crusts from the first section of dough and place them on the prepared baking sheet. Spoon 1 tablespoon of jam onto each crust and spread it evenly, leaving ½ inch (13 mm) of space at the edges.

8. Roll out the second section of dough and cut 8 more rectangles.

9. Use damp fingers to moisten the edges of the bottom crusts and place the remaining crusts on top of the tarts. Use your fingers and a fork to crimp the edges. Gently poke holes in the top crusts.

10. Bake for 18 to 19 minutes, until the edges are golden and the filling is sizzling. Let the tarts cool completely. Frost the tarts with Vanilla Frosting (page 294) or sprinkle them with Powdered Sugar (page 286), if desired.

(recipe continues)

TO FREEZE

Freeze unfrosted Toaster Tarts in an airtight container for up to 6 months. Thaw in the refrigerator; reheat at 325°F (165°C) for 5 to 6 minutes.

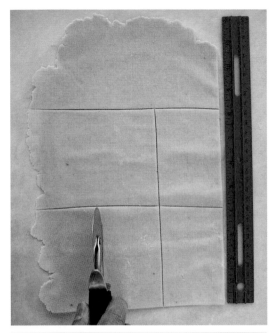

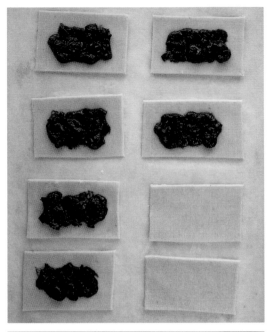

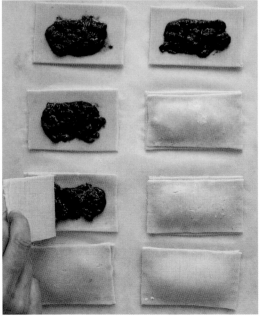

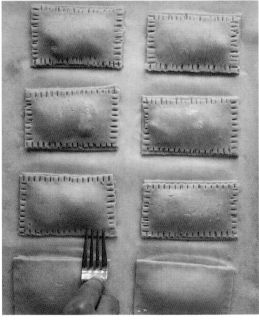

English Muffins

These muffins will get your day off to a great start, but don't save them just for breakfast; they can be a replacement for a sandwich roll and can also be used to make kid-friendly pizzas! English muffin rings help these to rise in the proper shape; if you forgo the rings your muffins will be a less traditional shape but still tasty.

400 grams (about 3 cups plus 1 tablespoon) Pastry Flour Blend (page 24)

1 teaspoon xanthan gum

2¼ teaspoons quick-rising yeast

1 tablespoon flaxseed meal

2 tablespoons organic cane sugar

½ teaspoon salt

3 teaspoons baking powder

1 cup (240 ml) plus 2 tablespoons Hemp Milk (page 31) or non-dairy milk of choice, warmed to 100°F (38°C)

1 tablespoon apple cider vinegar

3 tablespoons grapeseed oil

¼ cup (33 g) cornmeal

1. Line a large baking sheet with parchment paper. Place eight English muffin rings on top.

2. Mix together the flour, xanthan gum, yeast, flaxseed meal, sugar, salt, and baking powder in a medium bowl.

3. Blend 1 cup (240 ml) of milk, vinegar, and oil together in a large bowl, using a mixer on medium speed, about 30 seconds.

4. Slowly add the dry ingredients and mix on medium-low until combined. Increase the speed to medium-high and beat for 2 minutes. Add up to 2 tablespoons of milk as needed, ½ tablespoon at a time, until the dough is sticking to the sides of the bowl.

5. Sprinkle 2 tablespoons of cornmeal on a smooth prep surface. Lift the dough from the mixing bowl, form it into a large ball, and place it on top of the cornmeal. Use a bench knife (see tool tip on page 132) to roll the dough in the cornmeal and create a coated log.

6. Slice the log into 8 hockey puck–shaped pieces. Coat each piece on all sides with the remaining cornmeal and place them in the English muffin rings.

7. Sprinkle a few drops of water on a second piece of parchment and place it on top of the muffins (sprinkled side down). Place a second (smaller) baking sheet or cookie sheet (upside down), over the muffins and parchment. This will force the muffins to expand outward while they rise. If you are using English muffin rings, the second baking sheet will sit on top of the rings and parchment. If you forgo the rings, choose a second baking sheet with a 1-inch (2.5 cm) lip.

8. Let the muffins rise for 25 minutes in a warm, humid spot.

9. Preheat the oven to 375°F (190°C). Allow the muffins to rise for another 5 to 10 minutes while the oven preheats.

10. Bake (with the second baking sheet still covering the muffins) for 8 minutes.

(recipe continues)

11. Carefully flip the baking sheets over so that the top sheet is now on the bottom and vice versa. Remove the baking sheet and parchment that is now on top. Bake for another 7 to 9 minutes, uncovered, until the internal temperature is 200°F to 205°F (93°C to 96°C). The total baking time is 15 to 17 minutes. Let the muffins cool completely before slicing.

TO FREEZE

Muffins that you don't plan to use within 2 to 3 days can be frozen in an airtight container for up to 6 months. I recommend slicing them before freezing. Thaw at room temperature or in the refrigerator. Once frozen, English Muffins will be best toasted.

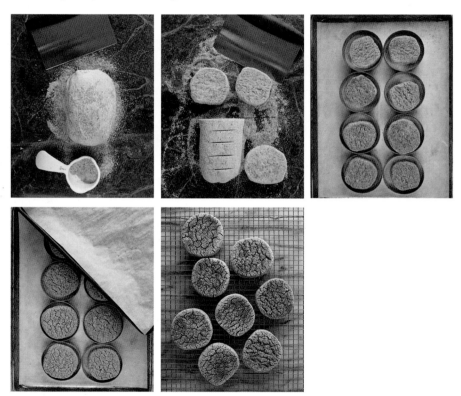

Bench knife

Also known as a pastry scraper or pastry cutter, a bench knife has flat sides with a sharp edge, allowing you to scrape, roll, coat, and divide dough. Use it on a smooth preparation surface when making English Muffins and other breads that require shaping. If you don't have a bench knife, use a spatula and a flat-edged knife to manipulate the dough.

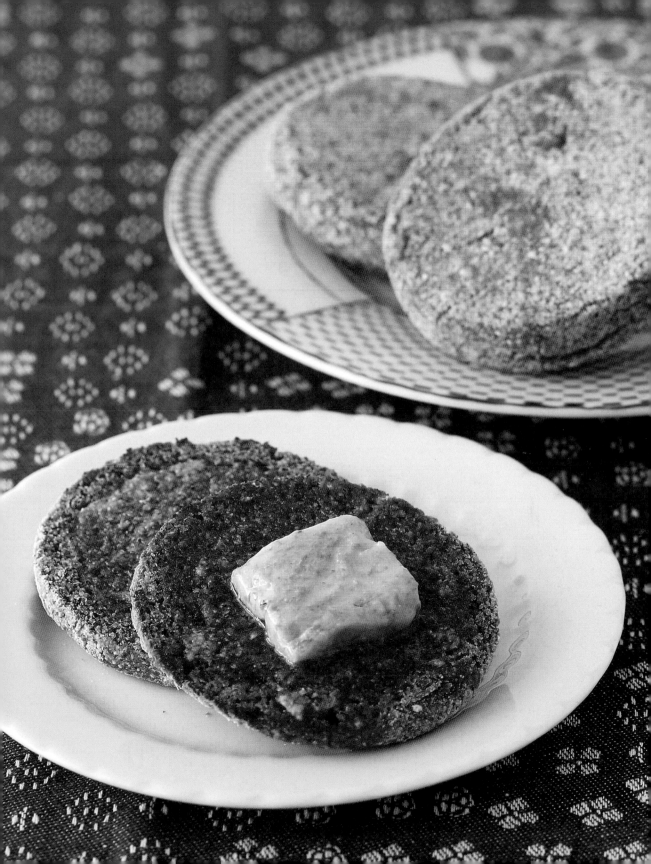

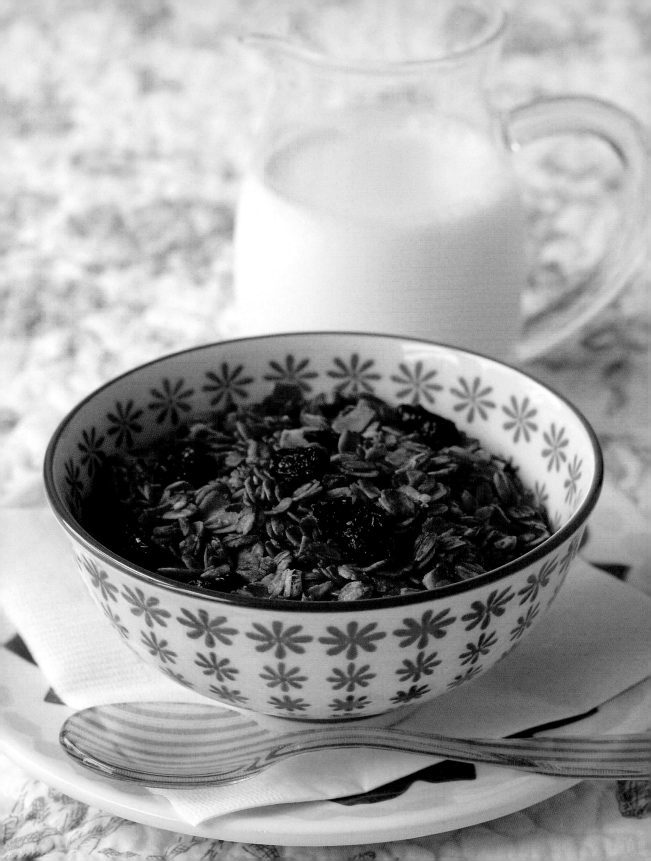

Cranberry Maple Granola

This recipe combines two classic New England flavors that I love—cranberry and maple. The trick to a crunchy granola is to cook it at a low temperature. It's easy to make but does require some elapsed time; I suggest making it at night for breakfast the next morning.

3 cups (288 g) gluten-free old-fashioned rolled oats

¼ cup (24 g) shredded coconut, optional

¼ teaspoon salt

⅓ cup (80 ml) pure maple syrup

4 tablespoons coconut oil, melted

1 teaspoon Vanilla Extract (page 288)

1 cup (120 g) dried cranberries

1. Preheat the oven to 250°F (120°C). Line a large baking sheet with parchment paper.
2. Combine the oats, coconut (if desired), and salt in a large bowl. Mix them together well.
3. In a small bowl, stir together the maple syrup, oil, and vanilla. Pour the mixture over the oats and toss all of the ingredients together until the oats are coated.
4. Spread the granola on the prepared baking sheet. Do not pack it down. Bake for 30 minutes.
5. Remove the baking sheet from the oven and stir the granola. Return it to the oven and bake for 30 minutes longer.
6. Remove the baking sheet again, and stir the cranberries into the granola. Bake for another 15 to 30 minutes (for a total of 75 to 90 minutes baking time) until the oats are golden and fragrant.
7. Let the granola cool and dry before transferring it to an airtight container. Store it at room temperature for up to one month.

TO SUBSTITUTE

To make a coconut-free version, leave out the shredded coconut and replace the coconut oil with another shortening (see page 7).

TO FREEZE

Freeze granola in an airtight container for up to 6 months. Thaw at room temperature.

Honey Blueberry Granola

MAKES 3¾ CUPS (430 G)

||||||||||||||||||||||||||||||||||||||||||||||||||||||||||||||||||||||||||||||||||||||||||||||||||||||||||||||||||||||||||||||||||||||||||||||

*W*ild blueberries are small berries native to North America. They have an intense flavor that shines in this granola. Crafted with honey and cinnamon, this granola smells oh so good as it's baking!

3 cups (288 g) gluten-free old-fashioned rolled oats

¼ teaspoon salt

½ teaspoon ground cinnamon

⅓ cup (80 ml) honey

4 tablespoons shortening (see page 7), melted

½ teaspoon Vanilla Extract (page 288)

¾ cup (100 g) wild blueberries

1. Preheat the oven to 250°F (120°C). Line a large baking sheet with parchment paper.
2. Combine the oats, salt, and cinnamon in a large bowl. Mix them together well.
3. In a small bowl, stir together the honey, shortening, and vanilla. Pour the mixture over the oats and toss all of the ingredients together until the oats are coated.
4. Spread the granola on the prepared baking sheet. Do not pack it down. Bake for 30 minutes.
5. Remove the baking sheet from the oven and stir the blueberries into the granola. Return the baking sheet to the oven and bake for 30 minutes longer.
6. Remove the baking sheet from the oven again and stir the granola. Bake for another 15 to 30 minutes (for a total of 75 to 90 minutes baking time) until the oats are golden and fragrant.
7. Let the granola cool and dry completely before transferring it to an airtight container. Store it at room temperature for up to one month.

VARIATION

For a nutty taste and even more crunch, add ¼ cup (36 g) raw, unsalted, shelled sunflower seeds in step 2.

TO FREEZE

Freeze granola in an airtight container for up to 6 months. Thaw at room temperature.

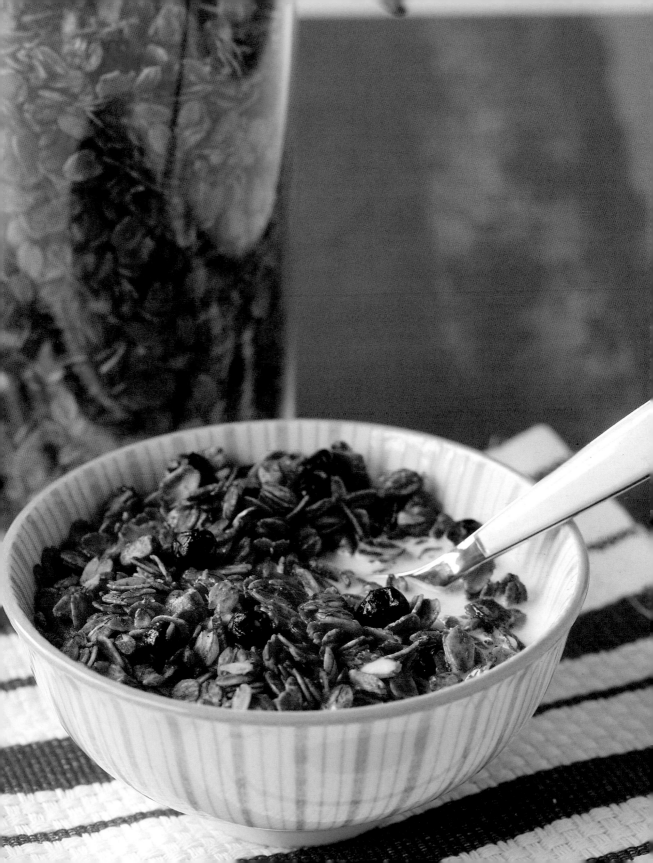

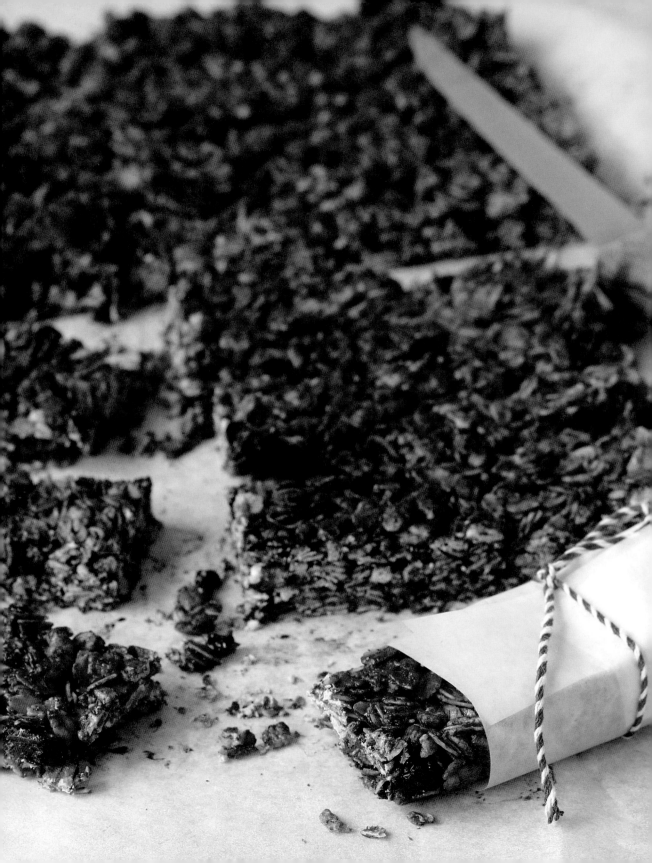

Chocolate Raisin Granola Bars

MAKES 16 BARS

||||||||||||||||||||||||||||||||||||||||||||||||||||||||||||||||||||||||||||||||||||||||||||||||||||||||||||||||||||||||||||||||||||||||||||||||||||||||||||||

*G*ranola bars are known to many as a grab-and-go breakfast, but they also make a terrific anytime snack. Feel free to vary the add-ins (or leave them out completely) to suit your taste and avoid allergens. Choose organic, unsweetened puffed rice cereal.

2¼ cups (216 g) gluten-free old-fashioned rolled oats

1 cup (30 g) gluten-free puffed rice cereal

2 tablespoons flaxseed meal

¼ teaspoon salt

½ teaspoon ground cinnamon

5 tablespoons shortening (see page 7)

⅓ cup (48 g) organic light brown sugar

⅓ cup (80 ml) honey

1 teaspoon Vanilla Extract (page 288)

½ cup (80 g) raisins, optional

½ cup (120 g) mini chocolate chips, optional

1. Preheat the oven to 350°F (180°C). Line a large baking sheet with parchment paper.
2. Spread the oats on the baking sheet and bake them for 5 minutes. Stir the oats, then bake them for 5 minutes longer (for a total of 10 minutes), until they are lightly golden and fragrant.
3. While the oats are toasting, combine the puffed rice cereal, flaxseed meal, salt, and cinnamon in a large mixing bowl.
4. In a small saucepan, melt the shortening, sugar, and honey together over low heat. Add the vanilla and stir until the mixture is smooth.
5. After the oats are toasted, reduce the oven temperature to 325°F (165°C). Line a

9 by 12-inch (23 by 30 cm) baking dish with parchment paper. Spray a thin coat of oil on the parchment, using a mister.

6. Add the toasted oats to the dry ingredients. Add the melted ingredients and stir until all of the oats are coated.
7. Stir in the raisins (if desired) and chocolate chips (if desired). Note that some of the chocolate will melt.
8. Spread the mixture into the prepared pan. Use the back of a spoon or a spatula to work it to the edges of the pan and pat it down. Bake for 18 to 20 minutes.
9. Let the granola cool for 10 minutes in the pan, then lift the granola (with the parchment paper) and transfer it to a cooling rack. Let it cool for at least 2 hours before cutting it into bars. Store granola bars at room temperature in an airtight container for up to 1 week.

TO FREEZE

Freeze granola bars in an airtight container for up to 6 months. Thaw at room temperature.

Polenta (Grits)

Polenta is extremely versatile. If you're eating it for breakfast, it's no harder to make than oatmeal—and indeed, it provides an alternative for those who can't tolerate oats. If you'd like to save some to chill and make Fried Polenta Sticks (page 160) or Polenta Croutons (page 67), you will need to cook it longer and add a few more ingredients (see steps 3 and 4). The additional ingredients noted are based on a full batch; if you plan to eat some for breakfast and save some to make Croutons or Fried Polenta Sticks later, modify the amounts accordingly.

FOR CEREAL

3 cups (720 ml) water

½ teaspoon salt

1 cup (140 g) polenta/corn grits or coarse-grind cornmeal

IF MAKING TO CHILL FOR FRIED POLENTA STICKS OR POLENTA CROUTONS

¼ teaspoon ground black pepper

½ teaspoon chopped fresh basil

½ teaspoon chopped fresh parsley

½ cup (120 ml) water

1 tablespoon light olive oil

To make cereal

1. Bring 3 cups of water and salt to a boil in a medium saucepan over high heat.

2. Turn the heat to low and stir in the cornmeal. Cook over low heat for 5 minutes, stirring occasionally. (Serve immediately with pure maple syrup and/or fresh fruit.)

To prepare for Fried Polenta or Croutons

3. Stir in the pepper, basil, parsley, and ½ cup (120 ml) of water. Continue simmering over low heat for 30 minutes, stirring occasionally. With 10 minutes left to simmer, stir in the olive oil. The mixture will become very thick. Let it cool for 5 minutes.

4. Grease a 7 by 9-inch (18 by 23 cm) baking dish. Transfer the polenta to the baking dish, smoothing to the sides. Let it cool for 15 minutes, then cover and refrigerate for up to 5 days. The polenta will solidify in the refrigerator.

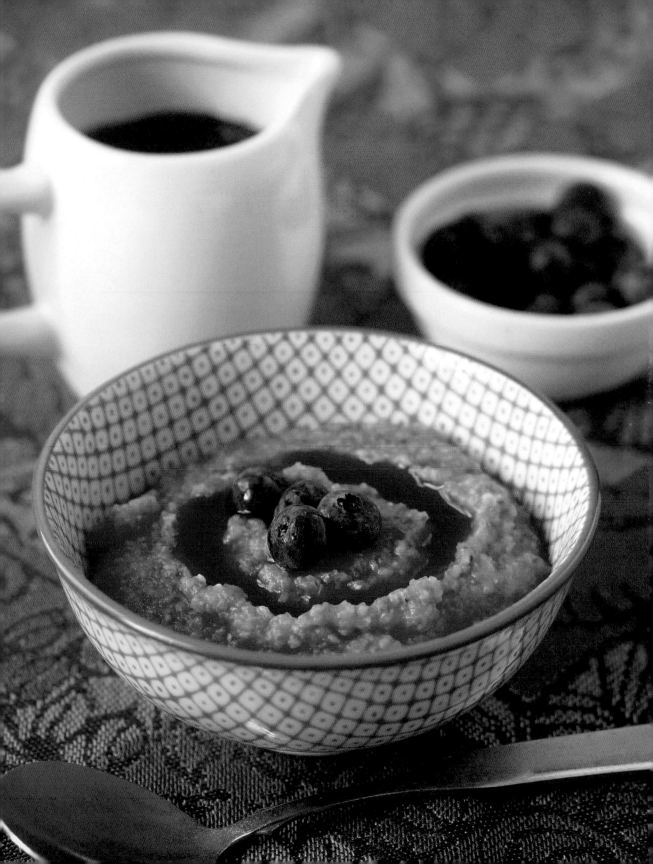

9.

Sides

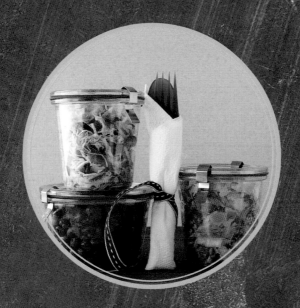

CAULIFLOWER CREAM AND CREAMED VEGETABLES ✒ POTATO SALAD

ASIAN-INSPIRED COLESLAW ✒ BAKED BEANS ✒ CAESAR SALAD

POTATO PUFFS ✒ FRENCH FRIES ✒ FRIED POLENTA STICKS

FRIED BATTER MIX AND ONION RINGS

It's impossible to be certain that the potato salad or coleslaw you can buy at the deli counter is safe from contamination. Likewise, it's no longer safe to fill up a container of tossed salad with beans and veggies from the island at the grocery store. Those of us with food allergies need to be diligent about selecting individual ingredients and washing produce well before using it.

Whether it's a dish to bring to the neighborhood barbecue or something to serve with the main course, this chapter has you covered with sides. Some can be tossed together without any baking or cooking (e.g., Asian-Inspired Coleslaw, page 151), whereas others require some elapsed time (e.g., Baked Beans, page 152), and still others require some diligent attention (e.g., Onion Rings, page 163), but all are delicious ways to complete your meal.

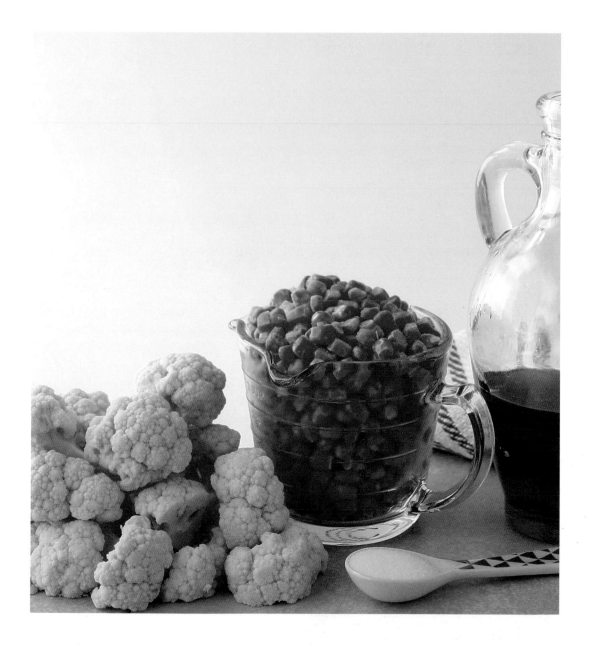

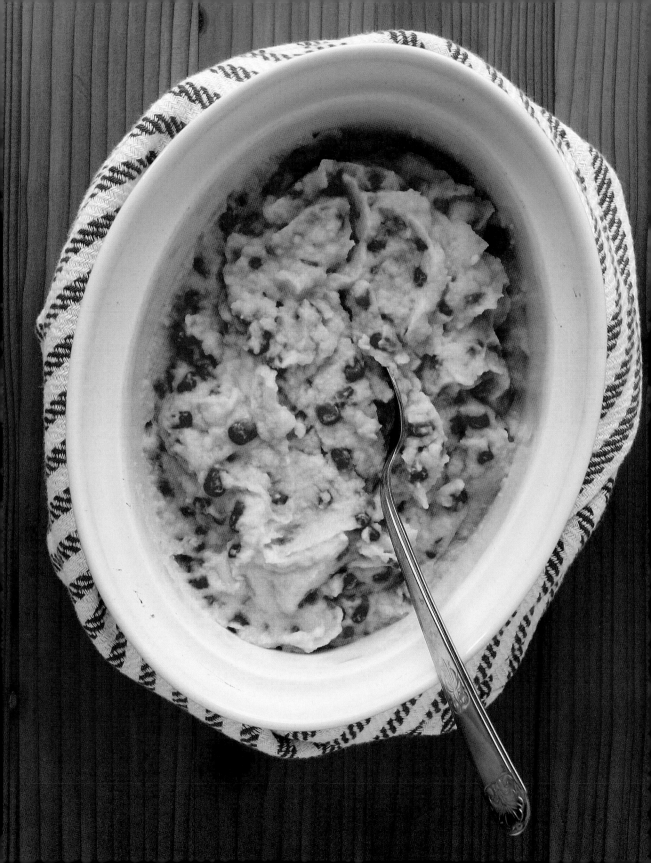

Cauliflower Cream and Creamed Vegetables

This simple recipe is an amazingly healthy way to make "creamed" anything—creamed corn, creamed spinach, creamed onions—whatever creamed vegetable or creamy pasta sauce you are craving, without a touch of dairy or even non-dairy milk. You are going to love this so much that you just might choose to buy a head of cauliflower each time you go to the grocery store.

FOR THE CAULIFLOWER CREAM

1 head cauliflower

2 tablespoons light olive oil

½ teaspoon salt

FOR THE CREAMED VEGETABLES

10 ounces (284 g) of your choice of vegetables (fresh or frozen), steamed, boiled, or prepared according to package directions

To make the Cauliflower Cream

1. Clean, trim, and chop the cauliflower into florets. Chop larger florets in half or quarters to create uniform-sized pieces.

2. Fill a medium pot with 2 inches (5 cm) of water. Place a vegetable steaming basket in the pot and fill it with the chopped cauliflower. Steam the cauliflower over high heat until fork-tender, about 10 minutes.

3. Transfer the cauliflower to a food processor or blender. Add the oil and salt. Puree until a smooth cream sauce forms. If not using immediately, refrigerate the cream sauce, covered, for up to 1 week. Heat at 325°F (165°C) for 20 to 25 minutes prior to serving.

To make creamed vegetables

4. Transfer the warm Cauliflower Cream to a serving bowl and stir in the cooked vegetables. Store and reheat leftovers according to the instructions for the sauce alone.

TO FREEZE

Freeze Cauliflower Cream or Creamed Vegetables in an airtight container for up to 6 months. Thaw in the refrigerator. Reheat at 325°F (165°C) for 20 to 25 minutes.

Potato Salad

Friends and neighbors will have no idea that this allergen-free version of potato salad was made without traditional mayonnaise or off-the-shelf salad dressings. Instead, Flaxseed Mayonnaise (page 99) is used to make a salad with added fiber and essential fatty acids—and that tastes marvelous! Add some blue potatoes, if you can find them.

Even though this potato salad contains no eggs or dairy, be careful not to let it sit out longer than an hour; it's the potatoes, not the mayonnaise, that contain the bacteria that can make you sick.

10 to 12 medium Yukon Gold and Red Gold potatoes, with skins, cubed

1 teaspoon salt

About 5 cups (1200 ml) water

1 medium red onion, diced

2 tablespoons diced Dill Pickles (page 209), optional

½ cup (120 ml) Flaxseed Mayonnaise (page 99)

2 tablespoons chopped fresh dill

1 tablespoon chopped fresh cilantro

1. Place the potatoes and ½ teaspoon salt in a large pot. Cover with water and bring to a boil over high heat.
2. Lower the heat to medium and continue boiling for 10 to 15 minutes, until fork-tender but not falling apart.
3. Place the potatoes in a strainer and run cold water over them for 30 seconds to halt the cooking. Drain the potatoes well.
4. Combine the onion, pickles (if desired), flaxseed mayonnaise, herbs, and remaining ½ teaspoon salt in a large bowl. Add the potatoes and stir to coat.
5. Cover and chill the potato salad for at least an hour before serving. It will keep for 3 days in the refrigerator.

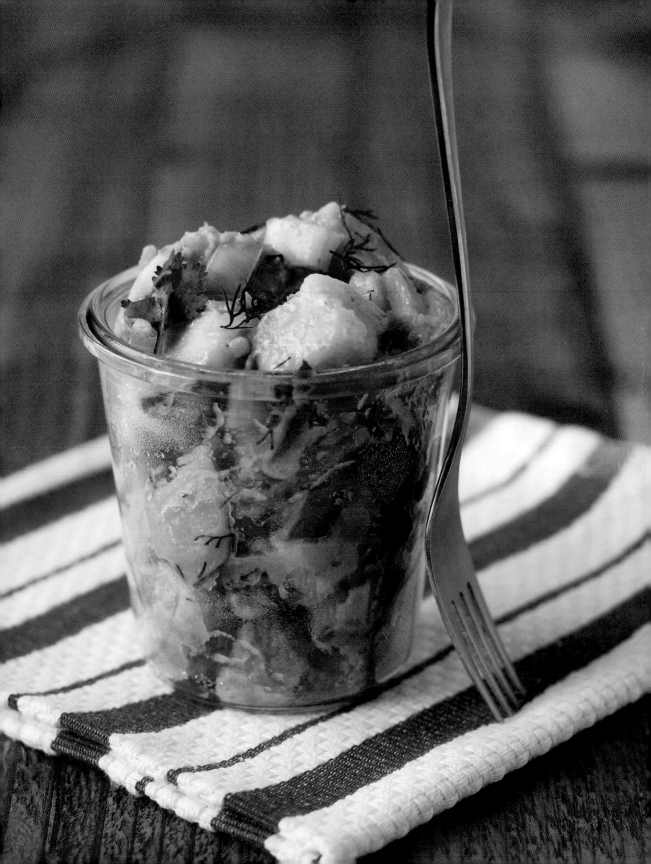

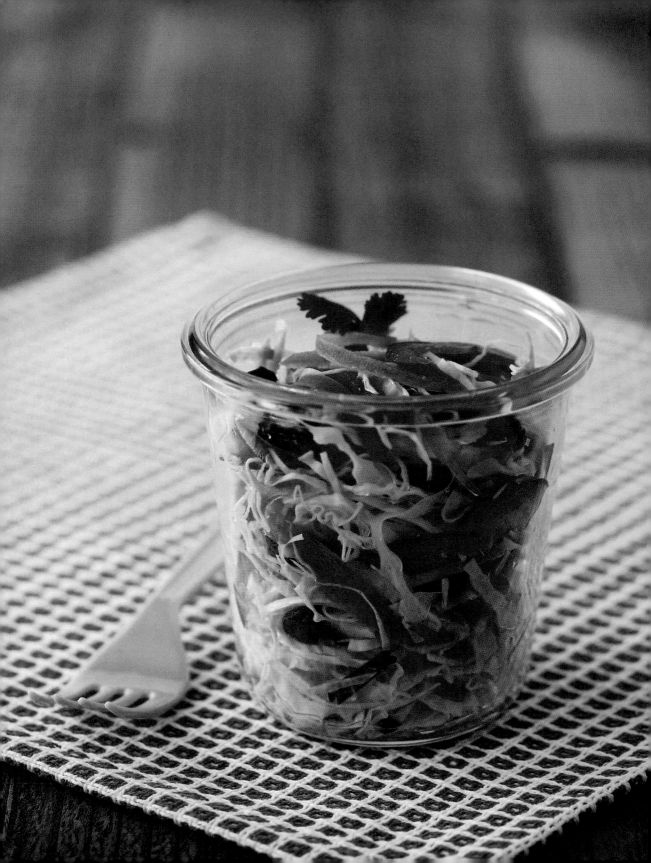

Asian-Inspired Coleslaw

This dairy-free and egg-free salad uses a tangy Asian-inspired dressing. Make it during the spring and summer months, when cabbage is in season, as an alternative to a traditional salad. This recipe can easily be scaled up for large gatherings.

FOR THE SALAD

1 medium head of green cabbage, thinly shredded

1 medium carrot, peeled and thinly sliced

½ green bell pepper, seeded and thinly sliced

1 tablespoon chopped fresh cilantro

½ cup (80 g) raisins or dried cranberries, optional

FOR THE DRESSING

3 tablespoons brown rice vinegar

3 tablespoons sunflower oil

1½ tablespoons organic cane sugar

1 teaspoon salt

To make the salad

1. Combine the cabbage, carrot, bell pepper, cilantro, and raisins or cranberries (if desired) in a large mixing bowl. Toss the ingredients well to combine.

To make the dressing

2. Whisk together the vinegar, oil, sugar, and salt until completely blended.

To assemble the salad

3. Pour the dressing over the salad and toss until coated.

4. Cover and refrigerate for at least 4 hours before serving. Coleslaw is best on the day it is made.

Baked Beans

In parts of New England, where I grew up, baked beans have somewhat of a cult following. I have a fond memory of my mother driving up to a small house, bringing an empty bean pot inside, and exchanging it for a new pot filled with the best baked beans—ever. I no longer have access to that small business source, but these Baked Beans rival that award-winning New England dish. Even those from Beantown will love them!

¼ pound (115 g) thick-cut bacon, cut into 1½-inch (4 cm) pieces

1 small onion, diced

1½ cups (360 ml) water

⅓ cup (80 ml) pure maple syrup

½ cup (84 g) Sucanat

¾ cup (158 g) Ketchup (page 95)

1 teaspoons salt

¼ teaspoon ground black pepper

Four 15-ounce (425 g) cans navy beans, drained

1. Partially cook the bacon in a large pot or Dutch oven over low heat, stirring occasionally, for 4 to 5 minutes, just to cook off some of the fat. Remove the bacon from the pot. (Retain all of the fat from the bacon in the pot.)

2. Cook the onions in the bacon fat over medium-low heat for about 4 minutes, until softened. Add the water and deglaze the pot, breaking up the brown bits, for 1 minute. Remove the pot from the heat.

3. Preheat the oven to 325°F (165°C).

4. Stir together the maple syrup, Sucanat, ketchup, salt, and pepper in a medium bowl. Add this mixture and the beans to the onions and water in the pot and stir them together well. Stir in half of the bacon. Layer the remaining bacon on top of the beans.

5. Bake, uncovered, for about 2 hours, until the beans are moist and tender and most of the liquid is baked off. Serve hot or cold.

6. Cool the beans completely before transferring them to airtight containers. Refrigerate for up to 5 days.

TO SUBSTITUTE

For a vegan version, omit the bacon. Cook the onions in 1 tablespoon of olive oil in step 2, add the water, and then proceed with step 3.

TO FREEZE

Freeze in airtight containers for up to 6 months. Thaw in the refrigerator. Reheat at 325°F (165°C) for 20 to 25 minutes.

A NOTE ABOUT USING DRIED BEANS

If you prefer to use dried beans, cover 2 cups (16 ounces/454 g) of dried navy beans with water in a large pot or Dutch oven and soak them overnight. In the morning, add more water (if needed) to completely cover the beans. Simmer the beans for 2 hours over medium-low heat, drain them, and then continue with the steps above.

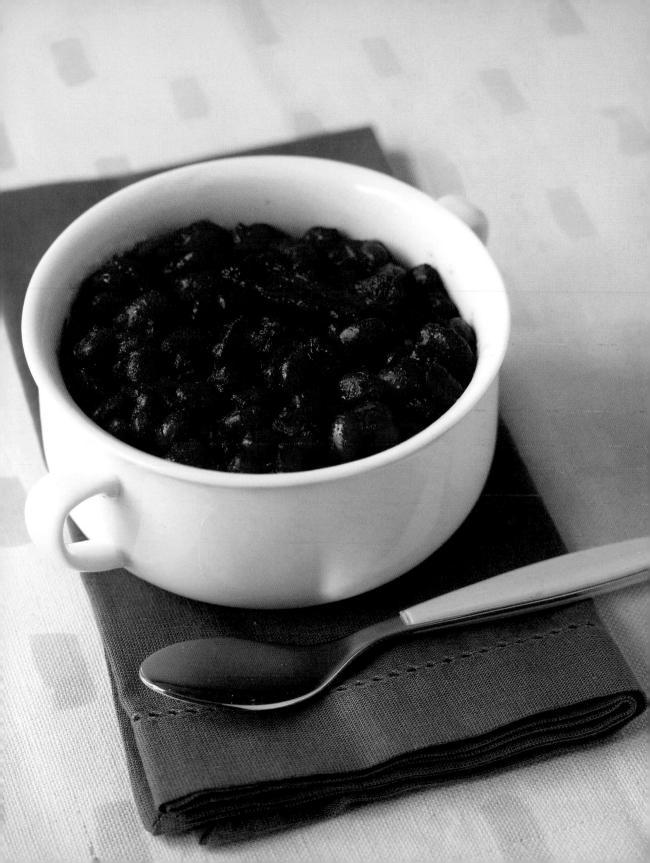

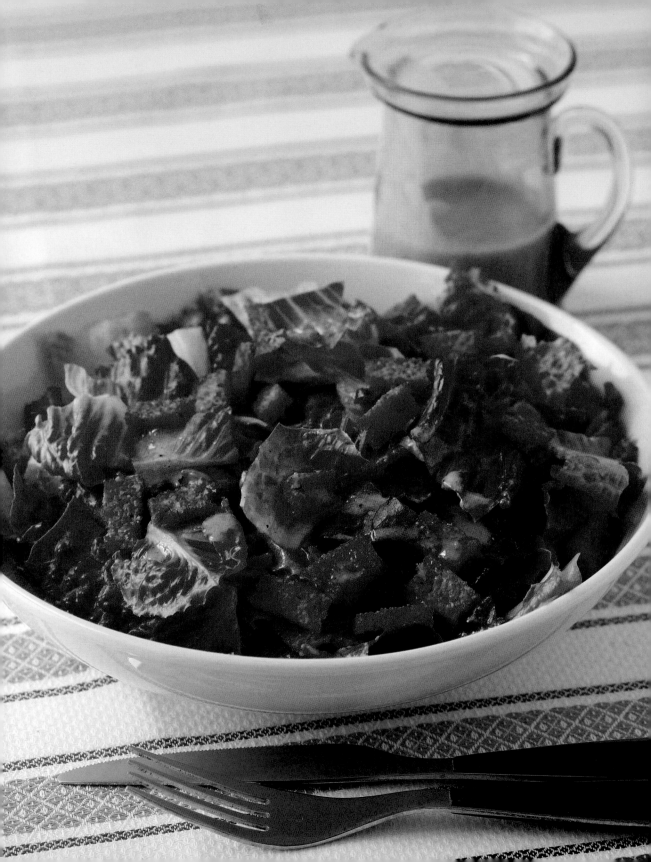

Caesar Salad

This salad combines Mock Caesar Dressing (page 106) and Polenta Croutons (page 67) with fresh romaine lettuce to create an allergen-free version of the traditional salad. There's no cheese, eggs, or anchovies here! Add your favorite protein to make it a meal.

1 head romaine lettuce, washed and chopped

½ cup (120 ml) Mock Caesar Dressing (page 106)

¼ cup (12 g) Polenta Croutons (page 67)

1. Toss the lettuce with the dressing, to coat.

2. Top the salad with croutons and serve.

TO SUBSTITUTE

For a corn-free version, Croutons made from leftover bread (page 64) may be substituted for the polenta croutons.

Potato Puffs

These pop-in-your-mouth puffs are a cross between a classic knish and a tater tot. Make a big batch and freeze some to reheat on the days when you are rushed to get dinner on the table.

3½ cups (525 g) russet potatoes, peeled and shredded

Cold water to cover

65 grams (about ½ cup) Bread Flour Blend (page 23)

58 grams (about ½ cup) corn flour

¼ teaspoon xanthan gum

1½ teaspoons salt

½ teaspoon ground black pepper

½ teaspoon onion powder

1 garlic clove, finely grated

¼ cup (60 ml) Hemp Milk (page 31) or non-dairy milk of choice

⅓ cup (80 ml) sunflower oil

1. Place the shredded potatoes in a large bowl and cover them with cold water. Let the potatoes soak for 15 minutes. Strain them and then squeeze them between paper towels to remove as much liquid as possible.
2. Preheat the oven to 350°F (180°C). Grease the cups of a mini-muffin pan.
3. Combine the flours, xanthan gum, salt, pepper, and onion powder in a medium bowl.
4. Blend together the garlic, milk, and oil in a large bowl, using a mixer on medium speed, for about 1 minute. Add the dry ingredients and blend for 2 minutes longer. The batter will be thick. Add the potatoes and blend on low speed to coat the potatoes with the batter, about 30 seconds.
5. Spoon the battered potatoes into the cups of the prepared mini-muffin pan. Bake for 30 to 34 minutes, until the tops are golden brown.

TO SUBSTITUTE

For a corn-free version, substitute 58 grams (about ½ cup) of millet flour or additional Bread Flour Blend for the corn flour.

TO FREEZE

Potato Puffs can be frozen for up to 6 months in an airtight container. Reheat from frozen at 375°F (190°C) for 15 to 18 minutes, or thaw in the refrigerator and then reheat at 375°F (190°C) for 7 minutes.

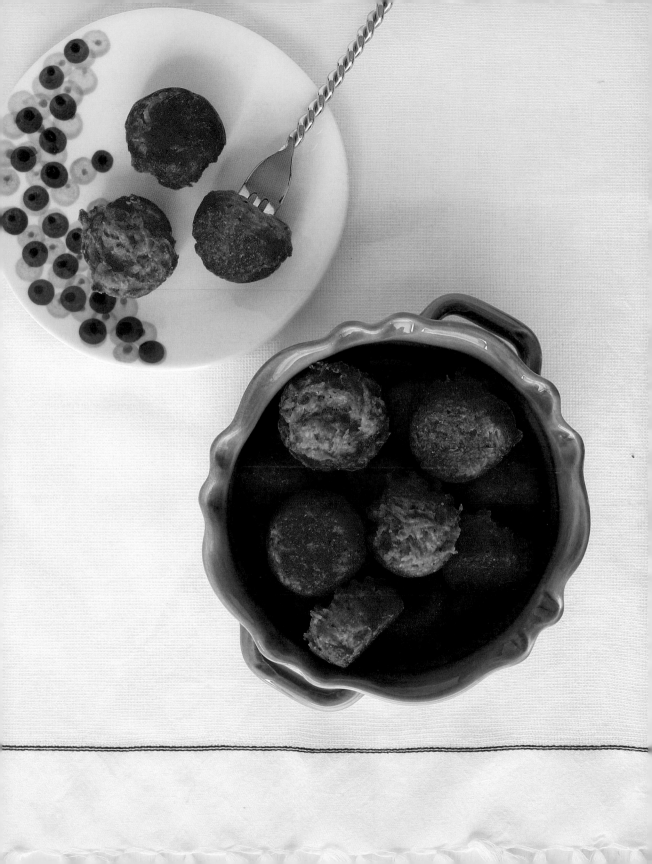

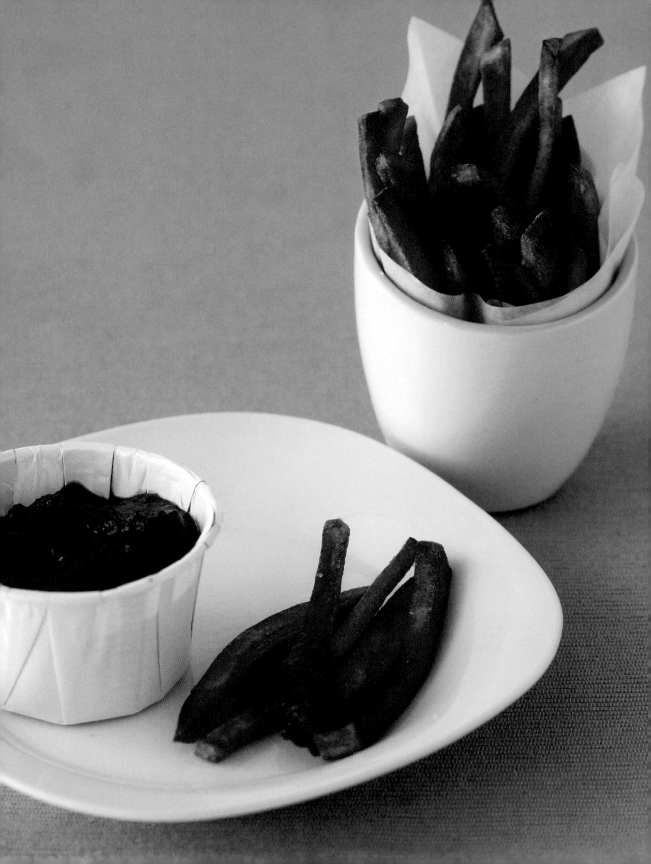

French Fries

The fryer at a restaurant or drive-through is usually a concern for those with food allergies. In some cases the same fryer is used to make all types of foods, often including those made with gluten, dairy, eggs, and seafood. In other cases the fries themselves are coated with flour—usually wheat flour. The best way to avoid these problems is to make fries at home. My favorite way to enjoy these is reheated after freezing; this will result in the crispiest fry!

3 large russet potatoes, peeled (optional) and sliced into sticks about ¼ inch (6.5 mm) thick

Cold water to cover

1 to 2 teaspoons salt

8 to 10 cups (1920 to 2400 ml) of sunflower oil (or high-heat oil of choice)

1. Place the potato sticks in a large bowl and cover them with cold water. Give them a quick swirl in the water to remove excess starch, then drain them. Soak the potato sticks for at least an hour in clean cold water and 1 teaspoon of salt.

2. Use a strainer to drain the potato sticks, then squeeze them between paper towels to remove as much liquid as possible.

3. A deep fryer can be used to make the fries, following the instructions for your fryer. Otherwise, use a medium non-reactive pan with high sides. Fill the pan with 2 to 2½ inches (5 to 6.5 cm) of oil. It should not be filled more than halfway.

4. Heat the oil over high heat. Try to maintain an oil temperature between 350°F and 380°F (180°C to 190°C). Watch carefully as you do this, and keep the kids away from the stove as hot oil can splatter and burn.

5. Work in small batches and use a heat-resistant slotted spoon. Add 4 to 5 potato sticks at a time to the oil until you have added between 15 and 20 sticks. The oil will bubble up rapidly as any remaining water boils off. Fry them for 2 to 3 minutes, until golden brown. Scoop them out using the slotted spoon and let them drain on a plate or rack covered with a paper towel. Repeat until all of the fries are cooked.

6. Optional: Fries made without a deep fryer may be softer than you expect. For crispier fries, follow these steps after frying: preheat the oven to 375°F (190°C) and bake the fries, on a baking sheet lined with parchment paper, in a single layer for 12 to 14 minutes.

7. Sprinkle the fries with salt, if desired.

TO FREEZE

Let the fries (prepared through step 5) cool completely. Spread them on a baking sheet lined with parchment paper and freeze them, uncovered, for an hour. Transfer them to an airtight bag and freeze for up to 3 months. Reheat the fries (from frozen) at 375°F (190°C) for 14 to 16 minutes, until they are warm and crisp.

A NOTE ABOUT REUSING OIL

You can save the oil used to fry French Fries or Onion Rings (page 163) and reuse it. Let it cool to room temperature, then strain and funnel it into a glass jar. Be sure to label the jar and use the oil only with allergen-free foods. When the oil smokes before reaching frying temperature, it appears dark and dirty, or your fries aren't crisping properly, it's time to replace the oil.

Fried Polenta Sticks

Instead of bread or potatoes, mix it up at mealtime with hearty fried polenta. This recipe takes advantage of Polenta (page 140) that you may have left over from breakfast and works equally well as an appetizer, side dish, or a special breakfast treat drizzled with maple syrup.

½ batch of Polenta, prepared for Fried Polenta Sticks (see page 160), brought to room temperature

1 tablespoon olive oil

1. Slice the polenta into sticks about ½ inch (13 mm) wide. Blot them gently between paper towels to remove excess moisture.

2. Heat the oil in a skillet over medium-high heat. Lower the heat to medium and add the polenta slices. Cook them for 2 to 3 minutes per side, until they are lightly browned on all sides. Serve immediately.

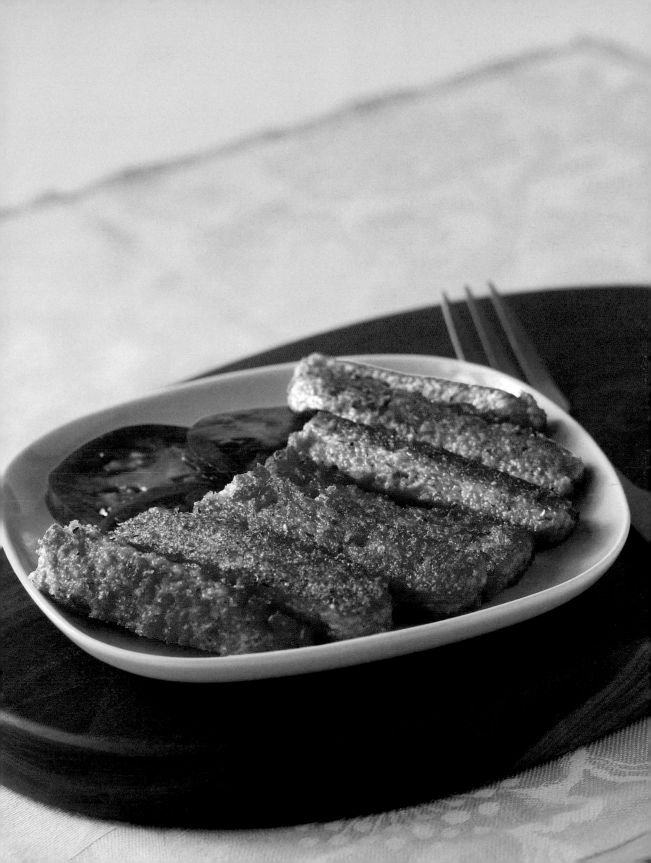

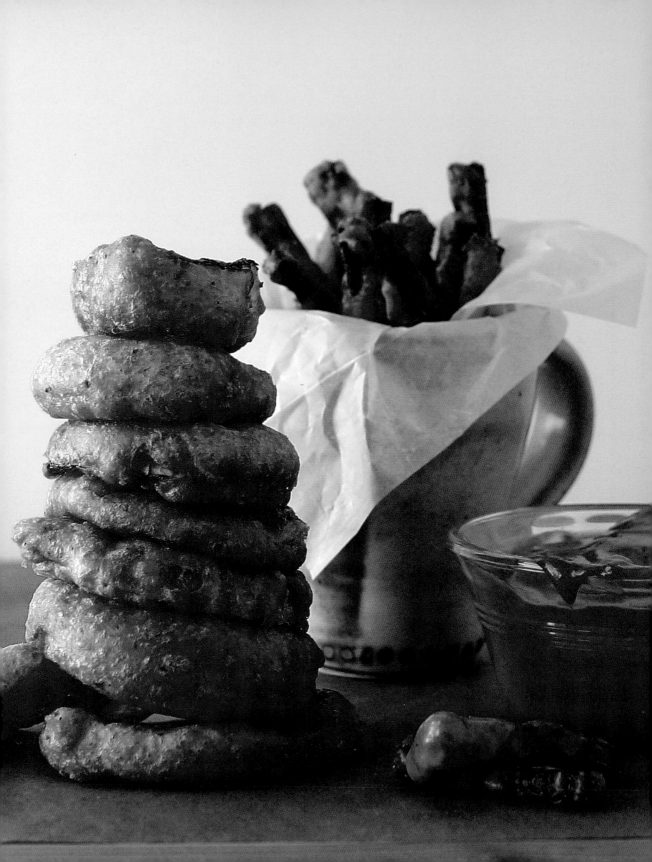

Fried Batter Mix and Onion Rings   MAKES 4 SERVINGS

*T*he garbanzo bean flour in this recipe, combined with seltzer water, makes the perfect batter for anything you've wanted to fry, including Fried Zucchini Sticks (see variation), and Onion Rings. Serve these homemade Onion Rings with Chipotle Mayonnaise (page 100) and you won't miss the chain-restaurant version any longer.

FOR THE BATTER

60 grams (about ½ cup) garbanzo bean flour

1 tablespoon corn starch

½ teaspoon baking powder

½ teaspoon salt

¼ teaspoon ground black pepper

1 Flaxseed Egg (page 42)

⅓ cup (80 ml) seltzer water

FOR ONION RINGS

1 large onion

8 to 10 cups (1920 to 2400 ml) sunflower oil (or high-heat oil of choice)

To mix the batter

1. Combine the flour, starch, baking powder, salt, and pepper in a medium bowl.

2. In a separate bowl, whisk together the flaxseed egg and seltzer. Whisk in the dry ingredients until well blended. The batter should be the consistency of pancake batter.

To make the onion rings

3. If you have one, use a deep fryer to make the onion rings, following the instructions for your fryer.

4. Otherwise, use a medium non-reactive pan with high sides. Fill the pan with 2 to 2½ inches (5 to 6.5 cm) of oil. The pan should not be filled more than halfway.

5. Heat the oil on high. Try to maintain an oil temperature between 350°F and 380°F (180°C to 190°C). Watch carefully as you do this, and keep the kids away from the stove as hot oil can splatter and burn.

6. Slice the whole onion to form ½-inch (13 mm) wide slices. Separate the layers to form rings.

7. Working in small batches, add 5 to 6 rings to the prepared batter, to coat them completely.

8. Add the coated rings to the hot oil using a heat-resistant slotted spoon. After about 2 minutes, use heat-resistant tongs to turn the onion rings over.

9. Cook for 1 to 2 minutes longer on the other side. Remove the onion rings from the oil and transfer them to a plate or a rack covered with a paper towel.

10. Continue frying in small batches until all of the onion rings are fried. If saving the oil for reuse, see page 159.

(recipe continues)

To make Fried Zucchini Sticks, slice 2 small to medium zucchinis into sticks about ¼ inch (6.5 mm) thick and 1½ inches (4 cm) long. Choose smaller zucchini rather than one large zucchini to minimize the water content. Working in small batches, add 8 to 10 sticks to the batter prepared through step 2, to coat them completely. Follow steps 7 through 10 to fry the zucchini sticks, cooking about 1 minute per side.

TO SUBSTITUTE

If you are allergic to corn, substitute another starch for corn starch. (I don't recommend substituting the flour in this recipe.)

10.

Pasta

and

Pizza

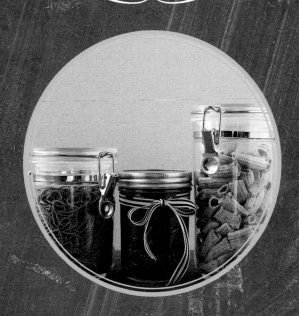

EVERYDAY PASTA ~ SPINACH PASTA ~ MACARONI

CHEESY SAUCE ~ PESTO ~ MARINARA SAUCE ~ PERFECT PIZZA

Pasta, pizza, comfort food. In this chapter you will find allergen-free and gluten-free alternatives for some of your favorite foods. Whether you are searching for one versatile pizza crust that allows you to send a safe slice to school on pizza day, or a sauce where you have control over all of the ingredients, you will find it here.

Making pasta from scratch is more time-consuming than opening up a box and boiling water, but there is nothing like fresh, homemade pasta. Don't rush home after a busy day at work and attempt to make pasta in 20 minutes. Allow some time and start the process in midafternoon to make fresh pasta for dinner.

Feel free to mix and match all of the recipes in this chapter. If you've never tried pesto on your pizza, here's your chance (see Pesto Vegetable Pizza on page 181). And of course, you have the option to choose an off-the-shelf pasta that is safe for your family; it will pair well with any of the sauces in this chapter.

MAKING PASTA

There are a few things you need to know to be successful at making pasta. Pasta dough is much stiffer than any other type of dough; very little starch is used and very little liquid is needed for the dough to come together. I prefer to mix pasta dough by hand because it allows the most control over the dough. When kneading pasta dough, you will need to work it hard (as if you were squeezing a stress ball). When mixed properly, pasta dough should hold together in a stiff ball. If bits of flour are falling from the dough as you work with it, add a tiny bit more water as needed (one teaspoon at a time); knead the liquids into the flour to make certain that they are well distributed.

Once the dough is mixed, shape it depending on the method you plan to use to form the pasta; if you are using an extruder (see tool tip below) or forming pasta by hand, pack the dough into chestnut-sized balls. If you are using a pasta roller, create large, flattened balls from the dough.

Homemade pasta is best cooked fresh and will cook much faster than the dried pasta you buy at the grocery store. In most cases you will need to boil the pasta for only 1 to 3 minutes: thinner pasta (e.g., spaghetti) will need about 1 minute of cooking time, whereas shells formed by hand may need up to 3 minutes (depending on how thinly you form the pasta). Always make sure the water is at a rolling boil before adding the pasta to the pot. When the pasta floats to the top of the boiling water, it is done.

Pasta-making equipment

A pasta extruder will allow you to create pasta in a variety of shapes. Stand-alone pasta machines, pasta rollers, or pasta attachments for a mixer will make sheets of pasta and allow you to make spaghetti. Keep in mind that a pasta roller or pasta extruder is the type of tool that is subject to contamination. I suggest reserving it for use with allergen-free dough.

Forming Pasta by Hand

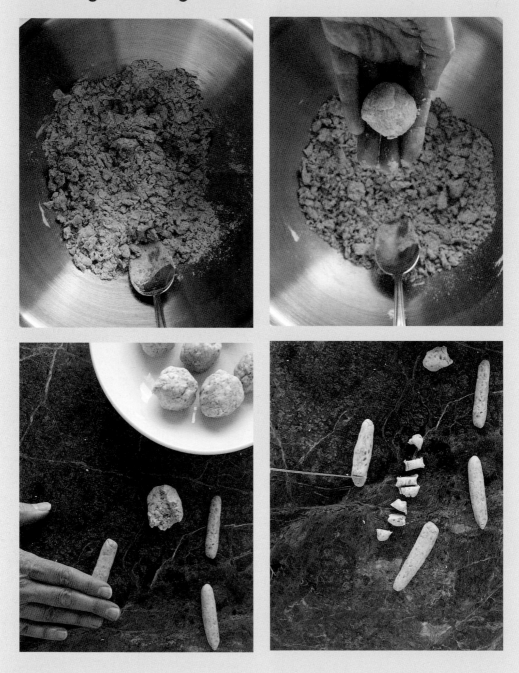

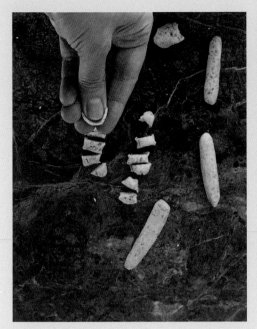 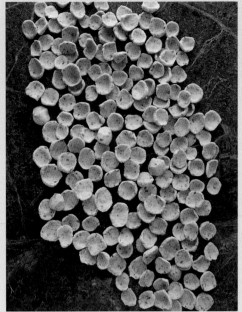

Pasta dough can be manipulated into shapes using just your hands. After forming the dough into chestnut-sized balls, cover them with a damp paper towel so they don't dry out, then follow these steps:

1. Pull off a small piece of pasta from the ball. Roll it between your hands (as you would with Play-Doh) to form a rope about ⅜ inch (10 mm) thick, then cut the ropes into ¼-inch (6.5 mm) long pieces.

2. **To make shells:** Roll each small piece between your fingers into a tiny ball and flatten it against your thumb. Curl the edges around the tip of your thumb to create a shell shape.

3. **To make gnocchi:** Roll each small piece into a cylinder. Use the tongs of a fork to make imprints in the dough.

If you choose to make pasta by hand, I recommend sticking to simple shapes, using your fingers and/or a fork. This is a great time to ask the kids to help!

Everyday Pasta

This basic pasta recipe uses flaxseed eggs as a binder and a combination of rice and millet grains to resemble traditional pasta. It can be made in any shape you choose. Double the recipe to feed a large family.

96 grams (about ¾ cup) brown rice flour

60 grams (about ½ cup) millet flour

32 grams (about ¼ cup) arrowroot starch

½ teaspoon xanthan gum

1¼ teaspoons salt

2 tablespoons light olive oil

2 Flaxseed Eggs (page 42)

1 to 3 tablespoons warm water, plus more for boiling

1. Combine the flours, starch, xanthan gum, and ¼ teaspoon salt in a medium bowl.

2. Combine the oil, flaxseed eggs, and 1 tablespoon of warm water in a separate large bowl.

3. Add the dry ingredients to the wet ingredients and stir them together until crumbly.

Test to see if the dough holds together by forming a small ball. Add up to 2 tablespoons of water as needed, 1 teaspoon at a time, until the mixture is stiff, yet smooth.

4. Form tightly packed balls from the dough.

5. Use a pasta machine or extruder, following the directions for your tool, to form pasta in the desired shape, or form the pasta by hand (see page 168).

6. Fill a pasta pot with water and 1 teaspoon of salt. Bring it to a rolling boil before adding the pasta.

7. Cook the pasta for 1 to 3 minutes. Drain, add sauce, and serve.

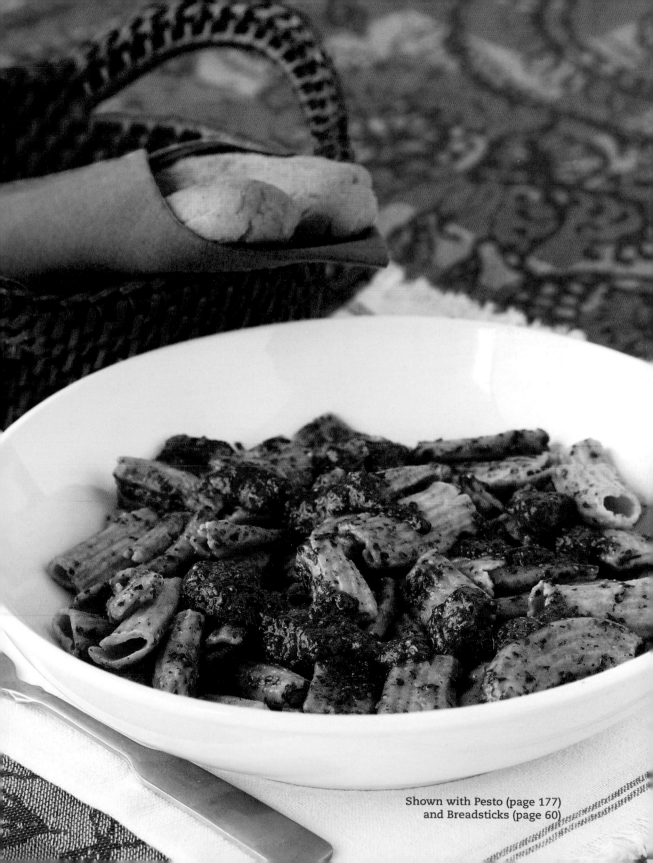

Shown with Pesto (page 177)
and Breadsticks (page 60)

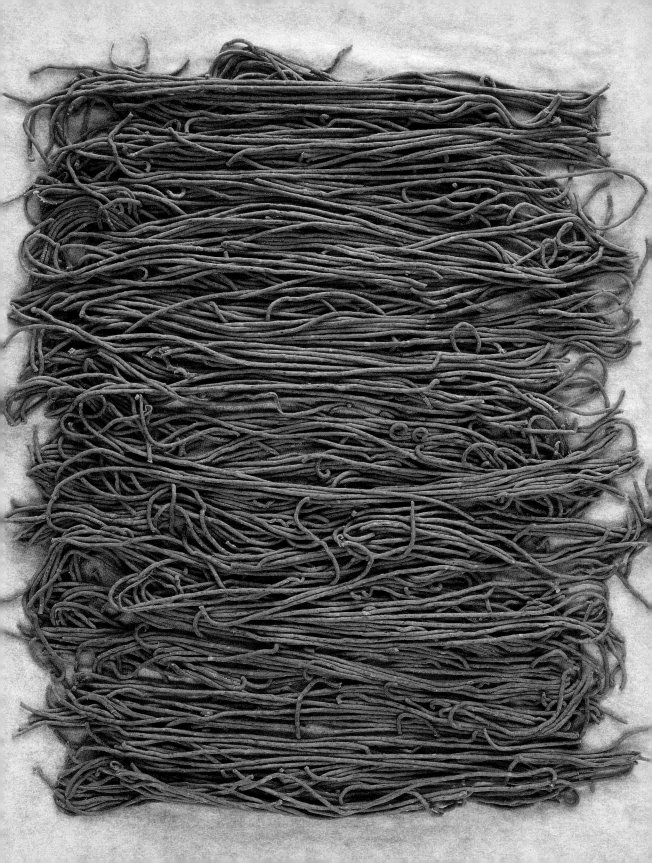

Spinach Pasta

Spinach adds fiber and nutrients to plain pasta. Cook some extra spinach for dinner and save some to make pasta the next day. Use about 2 cups (60 g) of fresh spinach to make ¼ cup (45 g) of spinach puree (see note below). Serve it with Marinara Sauce (page 178) for a colorful meal.

¼ cup (45 g) cooked spinach, drained

2 tablespoons flaxseed meal

2 to 4 tablespoons warm water, plus more for boiling

96 grams (about ¾ cup) brown rice flour

60 grams (about ½ cup) millet flour

32 grams (about ¼ cup) tapioca starch

½ teaspoon xanthan gum

1¼ teaspoons salt

2 tablespoons light olive oil

1. Puree the cooked spinach, flaxseed meal, and 2 tablespoons of the warm water in a food processor. Let it sit for 8 to 10 minutes. The mixture will be smooth and creamy.

2. Combine the flours, starch, xanthan gum, and ¼ teaspoon salt in a medium bowl and mix them together well.

3. Combine the spinach mixture and oil in a large bowl.

4. Add the dry ingredients to the wet ingredients and stir them together until crumbly. Test to see if the dough holds together by forming a small ball. Add up to 2 tablespoons of water as needed, 1 teaspoon at a time, until the mixture is stiff, yet smooth. The amount of water you need to add will vary based on how much moisture remains in the spinach.

5. Form tightly packed balls from the dough.

6. Use a pasta machine or extruder, following the directions for your tool, to form pasta in the desired shape, or form the pasta by hand (see page 168).

7. Fill a pasta pot with water and 1 teaspoon of salt. Bring it to a rolling boil before adding the pasta.

8. Cook the pasta for 1 to 3 minutes. Drain, add sauce, and serve.

TO COOK THE SPINACH

Steam 2 cups (60 g) of fresh spinach leaves with 2 tablespoons of water in a medium saucepan over high heat for 2 to 3 minutes, until the leaves are tender. If using frozen spinach, prepare according to package directions.

Macaroni

This rice-free pasta recipe uses sorghum and millet whole grains. Technically, macaroni is shaped in an elbow, but this recipe can be used to create pasta in any form—including hand-formed shells (see page 168). When tossed with Cheesy Sauce (page 176), this may become your child's new favorite comfort food.

90 grams (about ¾ cup) millet flour

64 grams (about ½ cup) sorghum flour

32 grams (about ¼ cup) arrowroot starch

½ teaspoon xanthan gum

1¼ teaspoons salt

2 tablespoons light olive oil

2 Flaxseed Eggs (page 42)

1 to 3 tablespoons warm water, plus more for boiling

1. Combine the flours, starch, xanthan gum, and ¼ teaspoon salt in a medium bowl.

2. Combine the oil, flaxseed eggs, and 1 tablespoon of warm water in a separate large bowl.

3. Add the dry ingredients to the wet ingredients and stir them together until crumbly. Test to see if the dough holds together by forming a small ball. Add up to 2 tablespoons of water, by teaspoon, until the mixture is stiff, yet smooth.

4. Form tightly packed balls from the dough.

5. Use a pasta machine or extruder, following the directions for your tool, to form pasta in the desired shape, or form the pasta by hand (see page 168).

6. Fill a pasta pot with water and 1 teaspoon of salt. Bring it to a rolling boil before adding the pasta.

7. Cook the pasta for 1 to 3 minutes. Drain, add sauce, and serve.

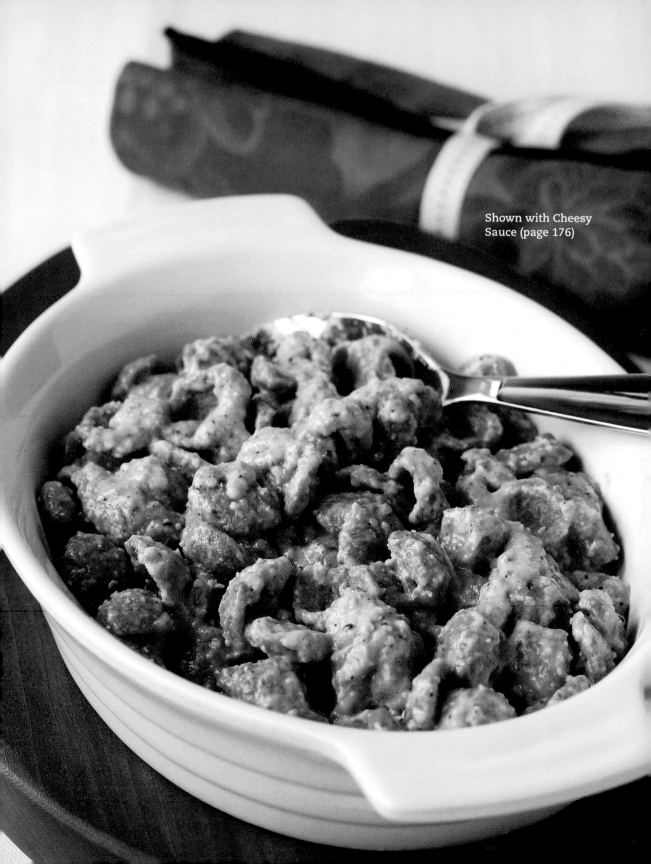

Shown with Cheesy
Sauce (page 176)

Cheesy Sauce

Shelled hemp seeds and hemp milk give this sauce a creamy texture and a mild cheesy taste; add some cheddar-style cheese shreds for an even cheesier version. The sauce mix is enough to cover two batches of macaroni or pasta. Refrigerate half of the mix and save it for the following week.

FOR THE CHEESY SAUCE MIX (TWO ⅓-CUP BATCHES)

½ cup (80 g) shelled hemp seeds

2 tablespoons corn starch

1 teaspoon garlic powder

½ teaspoon ground black pepper

½ teaspoon salt

FOR THE SAUCE (ONE BATCH)

2 tablespoons shortening (see page 7)

¾ cup (180 ml) Hemp Milk (page 31) or non-dairy milk of choice

⅓ cup Cheesy Sauce Mix

2 tablespoons Daiya Cheddar Style Shreds, optional

To make the mix

1. Combine all of the ingredients using a food processor or blender. Cheesy Sauce Mix (dry) can be refrigerated in an airtight container for up to 2 weeks.

To make Cheesy Sauce

2. Melt the shortening in a small saucepan over low heat.

3. Add the milk and whisk the liquids together. Increase the heat to medium and bring to a boil.

4. When the mixture just reaches a boil, turn the heat to low and whisk in the Cheesy Sauce Mix. Stir continuously until the sauce is thickened, about 1 minute.

5. Remove the sauce from the heat. Stir in the cheese shreds, if desired. Toss with pasta and serve immediately.

Pesto

Basil is easy to grow indoors, year-round, but August and September are when it's truly abundant. This no-cook recipe can be made in large batches when the sign at the CSA says UNLIMITED BASIL and frozen for use later in the year. It uses shelled hemp seeds in place of pine nuts and cheese to give the pesto a nutty flavor. Pesto can be used as a topping for pasta or pizza instead of tomato sauce or added to your oil of choice to make a dipping sauce for bread.

3 cups (72 g) fresh basil leaves, loosely packed

2 garlic cloves

½ teaspoon salt

1 teaspoon fresh lemon juice

1½ tablespoons shelled hemp seeds

¼ to ½ cup (60 to 120 ml) olive oil

1. Combine the basil, garlic, salt, and lemon juice in a food processor. Pulse ten to twelve times. Pack down the pesto leaves and scrape the sides of the bowl as needed, until all ingredients are chopped.

2. Add the hemp seeds and ¼ cup (60 ml) of olive oil. Puree for 20 to 30 seconds, until the mixture is smooth.

3. If you plan to use the pesto with pasta or for topping a pizza (see page 181), add an additional ¼ cup (60 ml) of oil. Heat the pesto in a small saucepan over low heat for 10 minutes, or until you are ready to toss it with the pasta.

TO FREEZE

Pesto can be frozen in ice cube trays; once frozen, transfer the pesto cubes to an airtight container. Use within 3 months.

Marinara Sauce

MAKES 4 CUPS (850 G)
Use two 1-pint (16-ounce/480 ml) jars if canning

*T*his classic sauce can be made with tomatoes from the garden, a local farm, or the grocery store—fresh or canned. If working with fresh tomatoes, choose a combination of round and plum tomatoes for best results. If you are canning, be sure to peel the tomatoes and add the lemon juice to the jars to reach the appropriate pH level (see page 73).

2 tablespoons olive oil

1 medium onion, chopped

4 garlic cloves, minced

3½ pounds (1586 g) tomatoes, peeled and chopped into large pieces, or two 28-ounce (794 g) cans whole peeled tomatoes

1 tablespoon chopped fresh parsley

¼ teaspoon dried oregano

2 teaspoons salt

½ teaspoon ground black pepper

3 tablespoons fresh lemon juice (if canning)

1. If you are canning, start boiling the jars to be used and follow the Steps for Canning on page 74.

2. Heat the oil in a large pot over medium-high heat. Add the onion and sauté for 2 minutes, until just softened. Add the garlic and sauté for 1 minute longer.

3. Add the tomatoes, parsley, oregano, salt, and pepper. Bring the sauce to a boil for 3 minutes. Use a potato masher to break up the tomatoes. How much to mash depends on how chunky you like your sauce.

4. Bring the sauce to a boil again, then reduce the heat to medium-low. Bring to a low boil, uncovered, and cook over medium-low heat for 20 to 30 minutes, stirring occasionally. How long to boil depends on how thick you like your sauce.

5. If you are canning, add 1½ tablespoons of lemon juice to each pint jar before adding the tomato sauce, leaving ½ inch (13 mm) of headspace, and process in a water bath for 35 minutes. Otherwise, let the sauce cool and then transfer it to airtight containers; refrigerate for up to 1 week or freeze for up to 6 months.

TO PEEL AND PREPARE TOMATOES

*Cut out the stem, remove any bad spots, and slice a small **X** in the bottom of each tomato. Use a slotted spoon to plunge the tomatoes into boiling water for 20 seconds, then remove them and plunge them into a large bowl filled with ice water. Peel the skins from the tomatoes. Quarter the tomatoes and use the tip of a paring knife to remove any excess seeds and water before chopping them.*

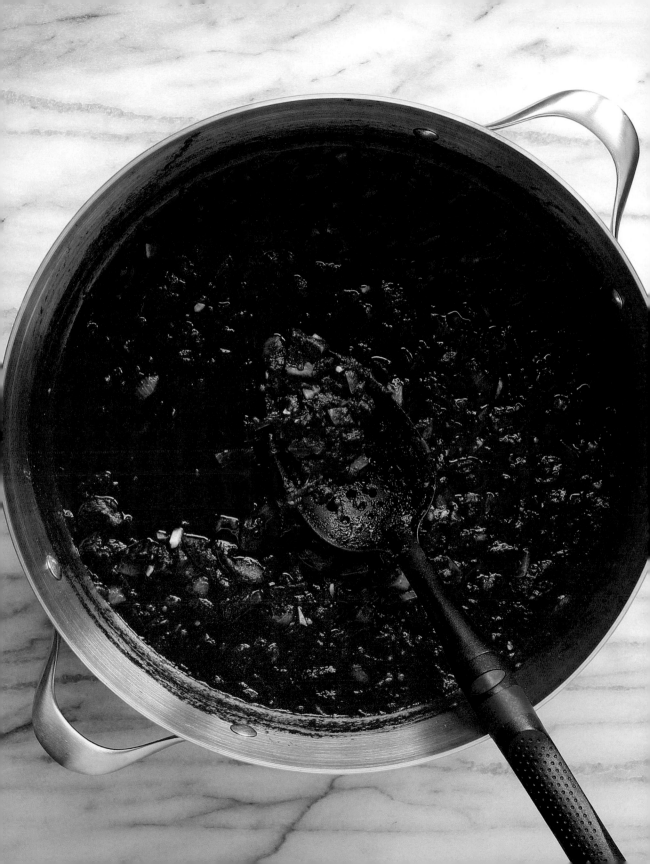

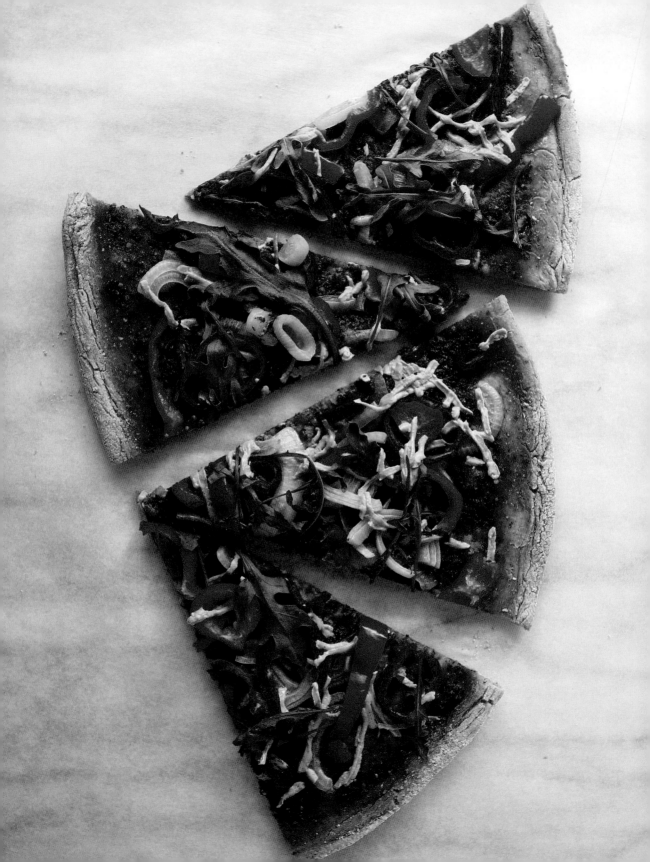

Perfect Pizza

Instead of picking up pizza on Friday night, make this crust at home. It's a thin crust perfect for holding your favorite toppings, whether meat or veggie. Make one large pizza to share with the whole family or two small pizzas—top one off for dinner and freeze one crust to save for later.

FOR THE PERFECT PIZZA CRUST

292 grams (about 2¼ cups) Pizza Flour Blend (see sidebar)

½ teaspoon xanthan gum

2¼ teaspoons quick-rising yeast

1 tablespoon organic cane sugar

½ teaspoon salt

½ teaspoon ground black pepper

½ tablespoon flaxseed meal

1 tablespoon chopped fresh basil or parsley, optional

2 tablespoons light olive oil, plus more for coating pans

½ cup (120 ml) plus 3 tablespoons warm water

2 tablespoons cornmeal or additional flour for dusting

FOR THE PESTO VEGETABLE PIZZA TOPPING

½ cup (120 ml) Pesto (page 177)

1 medium onion, peeled and sliced

1 medium green bell pepper, seeded and sliced

¼ to ½ cup (28 to 56 g) Daiya Mozzarella Style Shreds, optional

1 cup (22 g) arugula

Pizza Flour Blend
(292 grams, about 2¼ cups)

72 grams (about ½ cup plus 1 tablespoon) brown rice flour

68 grams (about ½ cup plus 1 tablespoon) millet flour

44 grams (about ¼ cup plus 2 tablespoons) sweet rice flour

60 grams (about ¼ cup plus 2 tablespoons) potato starch

48 grams (about ¼ cup plus 2 tablespoons) tapioca starch

Measure each flour by weight in a large mixing bowl (see page 22). Mix the flours together extremely well. Store the blend in an airtight container in the refrigerator for up to 6 months.

To *prepare the pizza crust*

1. Grease one 13-inch (33 cm) round pizza pan, two 9-inch (23 cm) round pans, or one 10 by 13-inch (25 by 33 cm) baking sheet.

2. Combine the flour blend, xanthan gum, yeast, sugar, salt, pepper, flaxseed meal, and basil or parsley (if desired) in a medium bowl.

3. In a separate large bowl, combine the oil and ½ cup plus 1 tablespoon (135 ml) of water using a mixer on medium speed for 30 seconds.

4. Add the dry ingredients to the large mixing bowl and blend on low to combine. Beat on medium-high for 2 minutes. Add up to 2 tablespoons of water as needed, ½ tablespoon at a time, until the dough is pulling away from the sides of the bowl.

(recipe continues)

5. Sprinkle 1 tablespoon of cornmeal or flour in the center of the pizza pan. Lift the dough from the bowl and place it on top of the cornmeal or flour. Sprinkle the remaining cornmeal or flour on the top and sides of the dough. Use a pastry roller (see tool tip below) to spread the dough to the edges of the pan, working from the center to the edges.

6. Proof for 25 minutes in a warm, humid spot.

7. Preheat the oven to 375°F (190°C). Allow the crust to rise for 5 to 10 minutes longer while the oven preheats and you add toppings to the pizza.

8. If you are making pizza crust to freeze and use later, see freezing instructions. If you are making Pesto Vegetable Pizza, continue with step 9. Otherwise, add your toppings to the pizza and bake for 16 to 18 minutes, until the toppings are done.

To make Pesto Vegetable Pizza

9. Spread the pesto on top of the pizza crust, leaving ¾ inch (19 mm) of space at the edges.

10. Layer the onions and peppers on top of the pesto. Add Mozzarella Style Shreds, if desired.

11. Bake at 375°F (190°C) for 16 to 18 minutes, until the edge of the crust is lightly browned and the toppings are sizzling. Top with the arugula after baking.

TO FREEZE

Partially bake the crust (without toppings) for 10 to 11 minutes at 375°F (190°C). Freeze in an airtight bag for up to 6 months. Thaw the crust at room temperature, add toppings, and bake at 350°F (180°C) for 10 to 12 minutes, until the toppings are done.

Pastry roller

A small pastry roller or rolling pin with a vertical handle is the best choice when you are making pastry, Mini Pies (page 258), or pizza crust—whenever you are rolling smaller crusts or you need to roll right up to the lip of a pan.

11.

Freezer Meals

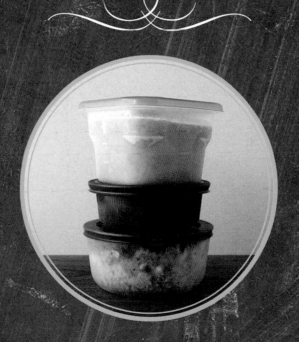

POT PIE WITH MOCK PIE CRUST ⌇ SHEPHERD'S PIE

CHICKEN TENDERS ⌇ QUINOA BOWL ⌇ FAJITAS WITH CORN

TORTILLAS ⌇ MEATLOAF ⌇ POTATO LEEK SOUP

Throwing together a quick meal or opting for take-out is not always viable in a household with food allergies. This chapter offers real solutions to mealtime madness, with dishes that can be made ahead, frozen, and reheated for lunch, dinner, or whenever you need them most.

In this chapter you will find family favorites that I have adapted over the years to accommodate food allergies, including a modified Shepherd's Pie (page 188), a Pot Pie (page 187) with a miracle crust, and a heartwarming Meatloaf (page 196). The ingredients are flexible, allowing you to accommodate whatever food restrictions your family has.

Whether you are preparing a meal for just one member of the family (while the rest of the family eats something more traditional) or you are cooking a safe meal that the entire family can enjoy, you will find plenty of options here. Bon appétit!

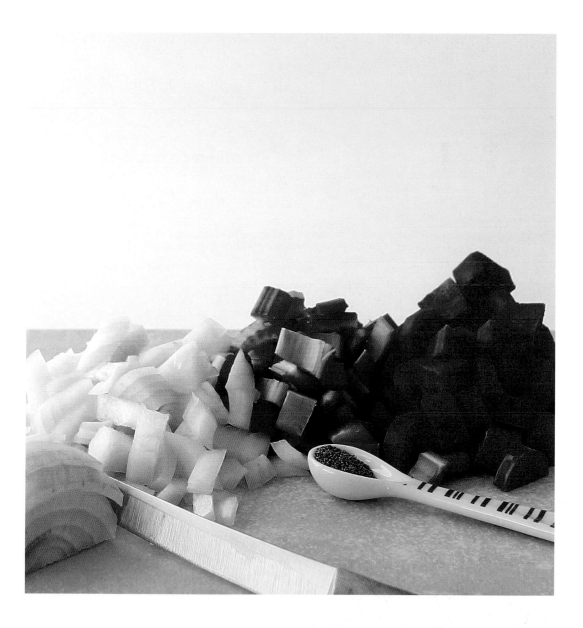

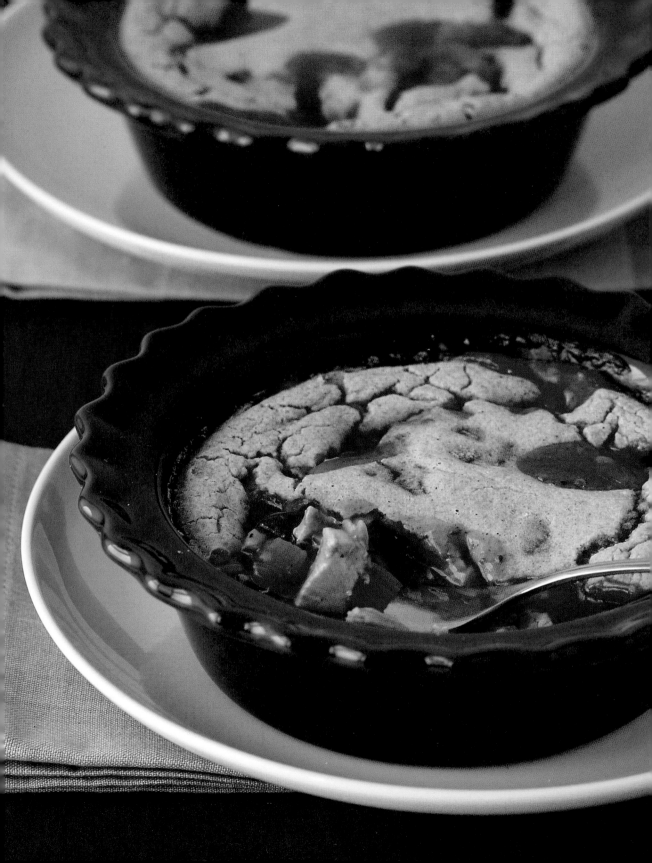

Pot Pie with Mock Pie Crust

MAKES 1 LARGE PIE OR 4 INDIVIDUAL PIES

This recipe includes a mock crust made from a simple batter that requires no rolling; the batter forms a crust around the pie as it bakes in the oven. Use this recipe with leftover turkey or chicken, or use the crust with any savory pie filling you prefer.

FOR THE FILLING

2 tablespoons olive oil

2 medium carrots, peeled and diced

2 celery stalks, trimmed and diced

1 medium onion, peeled and diced

3 cups (680 g) cooked boneless and skinless chicken or turkey, cubed (about 4 chicken breasts)

30 grams (about ¼ cup) superfine sweet rice flour

16 grams (about 2 tablespoons) tapioca starch

2¼ cups (540 ml) vegetable broth

½ teaspoon salt

½ teaspoon ground black pepper

¼ teaspoon celery seeds

FOR THE MOCK POT PIE CRUST

1 cup (240 ml) Rice Milk (page 32) or non-dairy milk of choice

3 teaspoons Ener-G Egg Replacer (page 41) mixed with 4 tablespoons warm water

92 grams (about ⅔ cup) Pancake and Baking Mix (page 24)

1. Preheat the oven to 350°F (180°C). Grease a 2-quart (1.9 L) baking dish, or four ½-quart (0.5 L) individual baking dishes.

To *prepare the filling*

2. Heat the olive oil in a large skillet over medium heat. Add the carrots, celery, and onions and cook for 3 to 5 minutes, stirring occasionally, until the onions are translucent.

3. Stir in the meat and cook for another 2 minutes.

4. Whisk together the flour, starch, and ½ cup (120 ml) broth. Pour this mixture into the skillet with the meat and vegetables. Immediately pour the remaining 1¾ cups (420 ml) of broth into the skillet and stir everything together well.

5. Add the salt, pepper, and celery seeds and cook for another 3 to 5 minutes, until thickened.

6. Pour the filling into the prepared baking dish(es). Leave ½ inch (13 mm) of head-space to the lip of the baking dish(es) for the crust.

To *prepare the crust*

7. Whisk together the milk and egg replacer in a small bowl. Whisk in the Pancake and Baking Mix. Pour the mixture over the pie(s).

8. Bake for 25 to 35 minutes, until the crust is formed and the filling is bubbling.

TO FREEZE

Freeze pot pie filling (prepared through step 5) in airtight containers for up to 6 months. Thaw in the refrigerator. Prepare the batter for the crust when you are ready to bake (steps 7 and 8); bake at 350°F (180°C) for up to 35 minutes.

Shepherd's Pie

Throughout my childhood I knew shepherd's pie as pâté chinois. My French Canadian grandmother taught me that this one-dish meal was intended to use up leftovers. I have since learned that Chinese cooks fed French Canadian railway workers the dish because it was inexpensive and easy to prepare. The workers brought the recipe with them to their home communities, including the small town in Rhode Island where I was born, and it has been a favorite in my family for years. Over time, I have adapted the recipe to use Cauliflower Cream (page 147) instead of potatoes.

1 pound (454 g) ground beef

1 tablespoon olive oil

1 small onion, peeled and diced

1 garlic clove, minced

¼ teaspoon salt

½ teaspoon ground black pepper

One 10-ounce (284 g) package frozen corn, thawed and drained, or one 15-ounce (438 g) can corn, drained

1 batch of Cauliflower Cream (page 147)

1. Preheat a medium skillet over medium-high heat. Lower the heat to medium, add the ground beef, and cook for 5 to 6 minutes, until the meat is no longer pink, stirring frequently. Drain the fat from the meat and set it aside.

2. Heat the olive oil in a small skillet, over medium heat. Lower the heat to medium-low, add the onions and garlic and sauté, stirring occasionally, until the onions are translucent, about 3 to 4 minutes.

3. Preheat the oven to 350°F (180°C).

4. Combine the ground beef, cooked onions, garlic, salt, and pepper. Layer this mixture in the bottom of a deep baking dish.

5. Finish assembling the casserole by layering the corn on top of the beef mixture and then layering the Cauliflower Cream on top of the corn.

6. At this point you can freeze the casserole for baking at a later date (see freezing instructions). Otherwise, bake for 30 minutes. Refrigerate leftovers for up to a week.

TO FREEZE

I recommend using a bowl that is both freezer-safe and oven-safe (otherwise, freeze in an airtight container and transfer to an oven-safe baking dish when you are ready to reheat). Freeze for up to 6 months. Thaw in the refrigerator; reheat at 350°F (180°C) for 30 minutes.

TO SUBSTITUTE

Any ground meat (e.g., turkey or pork) can be used instead of ground beef; use beans instead of meat for a vegan version. Any cooked vegetable (e.g., peas or carrots) can be substituted for corn. For a more traditional version of this dish, substitute mashed potatoes for the Cauliflower Cream.

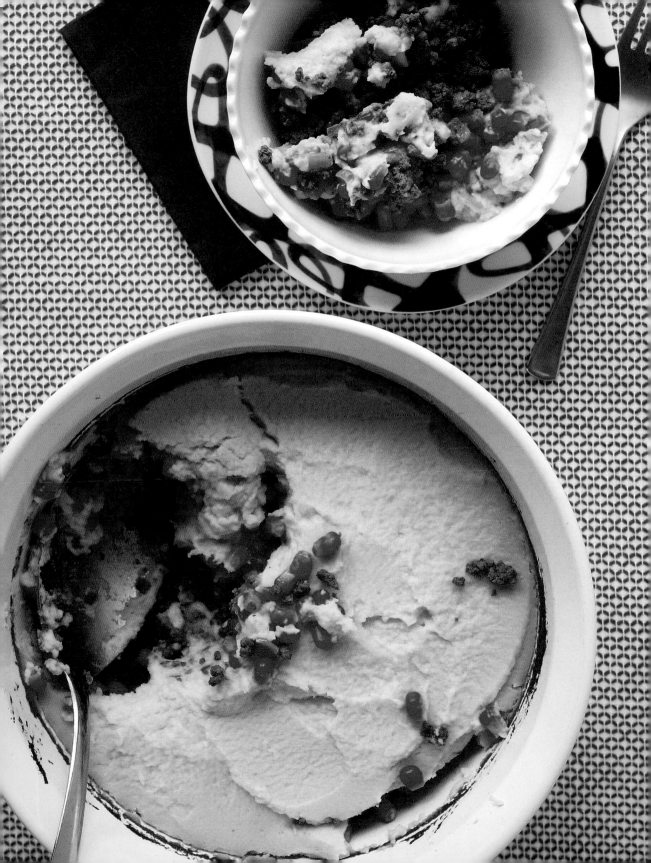

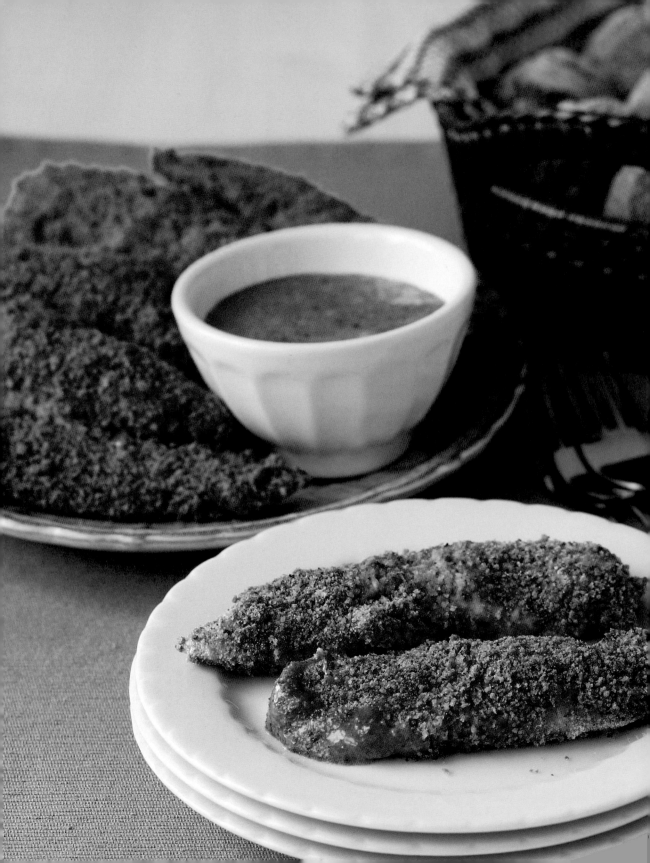

Chicken Tenders

Baked chicken tenders are healthier than fried chicken and tastier than traditional chicken nuggets. Make a large batch and store them in the freezer for a quick meal on a busy day. I suggest serving them with Honey Mustard Sauce (page 113).

64 grams (about ½ cup) Basic Flour Blend (page 23) or any individual gluten-free flour

½ teaspoon salt

¼ teaspoon ground black pepper

1½ pounds (680 g) boneless and skinless chicken tenders

3 Flaxseed Eggs (page 42)

1 cup (92 g) Bread Crumbs (page 63)

1. Preheat the oven to 375°F (190°C). Grease a 9 by 12-inch (23 by 30 cm) baking dish.
2. Combine the flour, salt, and pepper in a shallow bowl. Add the chicken tenders and toss until the chicken is coated with flour. Shake excess flour off the chicken tenders.
3. Place the flaxseed eggs in a separate shallow bowl, and the bread crumbs on a shallow plate.
4. Dip each floured tender into the flaxseed egg to create a moist layer, then roll it in the bread crumbs to coat it on all sides.
5. Place the chicken in the prepared baking dish. Bake, uncovered, for 20 to 25 minutes, until the tenders are golden brown and cooked through. Baking time will vary based on the thickness of the chicken tenders.

TO FREEZE

Freeze cooked Chicken Tenders for up to 6 months in an airtight container. Thaw in the refrigerator and reheat at 325°F (165°C) for 20 to 25 minutes, or reheat from frozen at 375°F (190°C) for 16 to 18 minutes.

Quinoa Bowl

The beauty of a "bowl" meal is that it can be prepared with just about any grain and just about any vegetables and/or protein, making this a very flexible recipe for those with multiple food allergies. I have chosen to combine quinoa with carrots and broccoli, and I added some garbanzo beans for protein.

To create your own version of this recipe, start with your favorite safe grain—brown rice, quinoa, buckwheat, and millet all work well. Sauté or steam some vegetables and layer them on top of the grain. Add some cooked meat, beans, or another protein, if desired.

1 cup (184 g) whole grain quinoa

½ tablespoon chopped fresh parsley

1 teaspoon salt

2 cups (425 g) cooked chickpeas (garbanzo beans), drained (or one 15- to 16-ounce/425 g can chickpeas, drained)

2 tablespoons olive oil

1 garlic clove, minced

1 large carrot, peeled and thinly sliced

1 small onion, peeled and chopped

2 cups (160 g) broccoli florets, larger pieces chopped

¼ teaspoon ground black pepper

1 teaspoon fresh lemon juice

1. Prepare the quinoa according to package instructions. Stir in the parsley and ½ teaspoon of the salt. Let it sit for 15 minutes. Meanwhile, continue preparing the additional ingredients.

2. Heat the chickpeas in a small saucepan over low heat. Let them simmer while you prepare the vegetables.

3. Heat 1 tablespoon of olive oil in a skillet over medium heat. Add the garlic, carrots, onions, and ¼ teaspoon of the salt. Sauté until the carrots are fork-tender, about 6 minutes. Transfer the vegetables to a prep bowl.

4. Wipe the skillet clean and return it to the stove. Add the broccoli, pepper, and more oil (if needed). Sauté until the broccoli is bright green, about 2 minutes. Add the lemon juice and sauté for 30 seconds longer.

5. Assemble the bowls for serving and/or freezing. Layer or arrange the ingredients, as desired, in the serving bowls. Add more salt to taste.

TO FREEZE

I recommend using ½-quart (0.5 liter) bowls or baking dishes that are both freezer-safe and oven-safe (otherwise freeze in airtight containers and transfer to an oven-safe bowl when you are ready to reheat). Freeze for up to 6 months. Thaw in the refrigerator; reheat at 325°F (165°C) for 25 to 28 minutes.

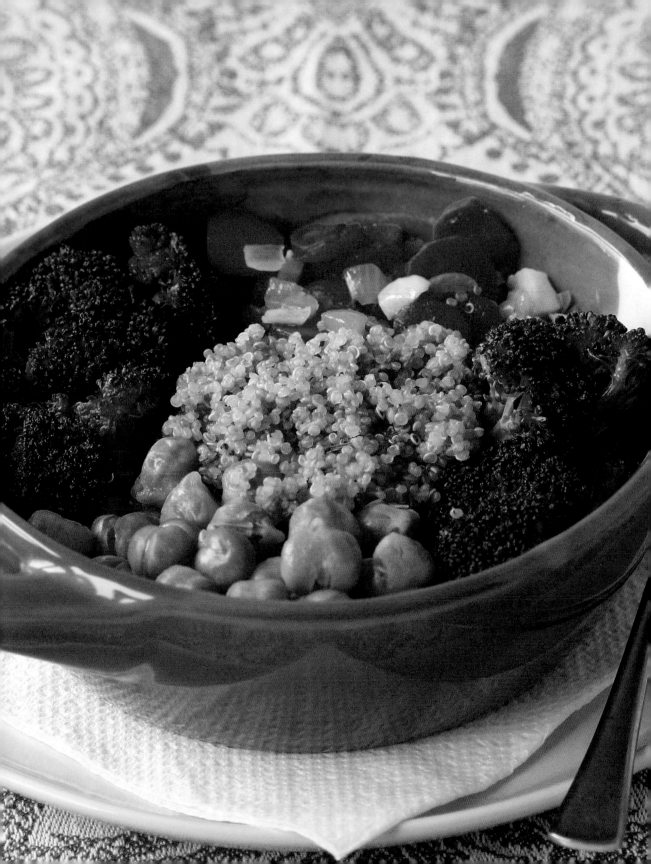

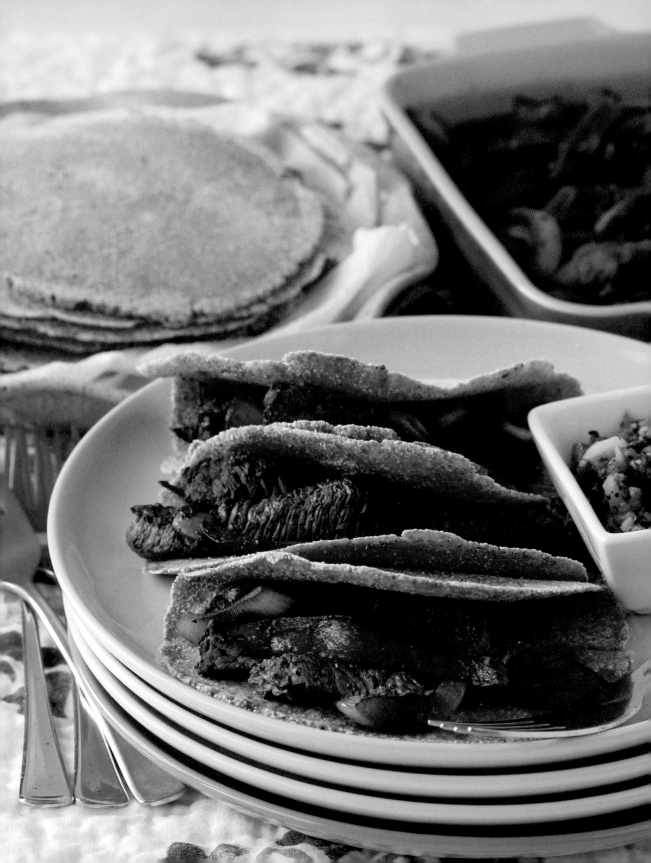

Fajitas with Corn Tortillas

MAKES 10 FAJITAS, 5 SERVINGS

he soft corn tortillas used in this fajita recipe are made with 100 percent corn—just like the ones traditional Mexican restaurants use. Make the fajitas with steak, as I have done here, or choose another protein. For a vegetarian version, try portobello mushrooms. You can also use these tortillas to make tacos or burritos. Top them with Daiya Mozzarella Style Shreds, if desired.

FOR THE TORTILLAS

232 grams (about 2 cups) masa harina, plus up to 2 tablespoons for dusting

¼ teaspoon salt

1 cup plus 1 tablespoon (255 ml) warm water

FOR THE FAJITAS

10 ounces (280 g) cooked steak

1 tablespoon olive oil

1 medium green bell pepper, seeded and sliced

1 medium onion, peeled, halved, and sliced

1 garlic clove, finely grated

2 tablespoons chopped fresh cilantro

½ teaspoon salt

½ teaspoon ground black pepper

To make the tortillas

1. Mix together the masa harina, salt, and water in a large mixing bowl, by hand, until the dough is soft and pliable. Separate the dough and form 10 tightly packed balls about 1½ inches (4 cm) in diameter.

2. Heat a large, dry skillet over medium-high heat.

3. Roll out each ball into a thin tortilla (about 6 inches/15 cm in diameter) between two sheets of parchment paper, using additional flour as needed to avoid sticking. Roll as thinly as you can. Use a cutter to create 6-inch (15 cm) rounds, or keep them freeform.

4. Cook each tortilla in the skillet, about 30 to 45 seconds per side.

5. Keep the cooked tortillas moist between damp paper towels until you are ready to assemble the fajitas.

To make the fajitas

6. Cut the cooked steak into strips and set it aside.

7. Heat the olive oil in a large skillet over medium-high heat. Lower the heat to medium. Add the bell pepper and onion and cook until the vegetables are just crisp and lightly browned, about 3 minutes.

8. Stir in the garlic, cilantro, salt, pepper, and cooked steak. Heat for 2 to 3 minutes longer.

9. Assemble the fajitas and serve.

TO FREEZE

Freeze corn tortillas (unfilled) in airtight bags for up to 3 months. Thaw at room temperature. Reheat up to 3 tortillas at a time, for 20 seconds per tortilla, between damp paper towels in the microwave. Freeze fajita filling in an airtight container for up to 6 months. Thaw in the refrigerator. Reheat at 350°F (180°C) for 20 to 25 minutes.

Meatloaf

Dressed up or dressed down, meatloaf can be served for a dinner party or an everyday family meal. This same recipe can be used to make meatballs to serve with your favorite pasta (see variation).

¾ cup (70 g) Bread Crumbs (page 63)

½ teaspoon salt

½ teaspoon ground black pepper

1½ tablespoons flaxseed meal

1 teaspoon chopped fresh basil

1 teaspoon chopped fresh cilantro

1½ pounds (680 g) ground beef

1½ tablespoons light olive oil

½ cup plus 2 tablespoons (150 ml) Hemp Milk (page 31) or non-dairy milk of choice

1 small onion, peeled and minced

1 clove garlic, finely grated

1. Preheat the oven to 350°F (180°C). Grease a 9 by 5-inch (23 by 13 cm) loaf pan.
2. Combine the bread crumbs, salt, pepper, flaxseed meal, basil, and cilantro in a large mixing bowl. Add the meat, oil, milk, onion, and garlic. Use your hands to massage the ingredients together until they are evenly distributed and the mixture is smooth.
3. Scoop the meatloaf into the prepared loaf pan. Pat it down evenly and smoothly to the edges of the pan.
4. Cover with aluminum foil and bake for 45 minutes. Remove the foil and bake for 15 to 25 minutes longer, until the meatloaf is nicely browned and pulling away from the edges of the pan. Let it sit for 10 minutes before slicing.

TO SUBSTITUTE

Substitute ground turkey, ground veal, or any combination for the ground beef. If you need to avoid flaxseeds, add an additional tablespoon of olive oil in place of the flaxseed meal.

TO FREEZE

Freeze in an airtight container for up to 6 months. I recommend slicing and freezing portions separately. Thaw in the refrigerator and reheat at 325°F (165°C), covered, for 25 to 35 minutes.

VARIATION

To make Meatballs: Coat the bottom of a large stockpot or Dutch oven with Marinara Sauce (page 178—you will need about ½ batch, or one 16-ounce/425 g jar). Prepare the mixture through step 2, then use your hands to form meatballs, each about 1½ inches (4 cm) round. Place the meatballs in the pot and cover with more sauce. Simmer, covered, over medium-low heat for an hour, gently stirring occasionally. Turn the heat to the lowest setting and simmer for another hour, or until you are ready to serve.

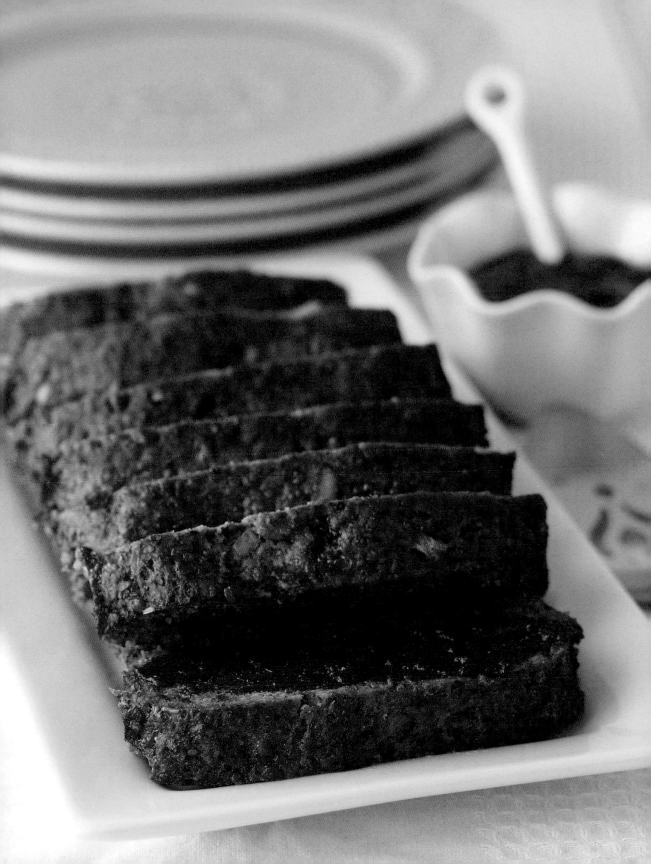

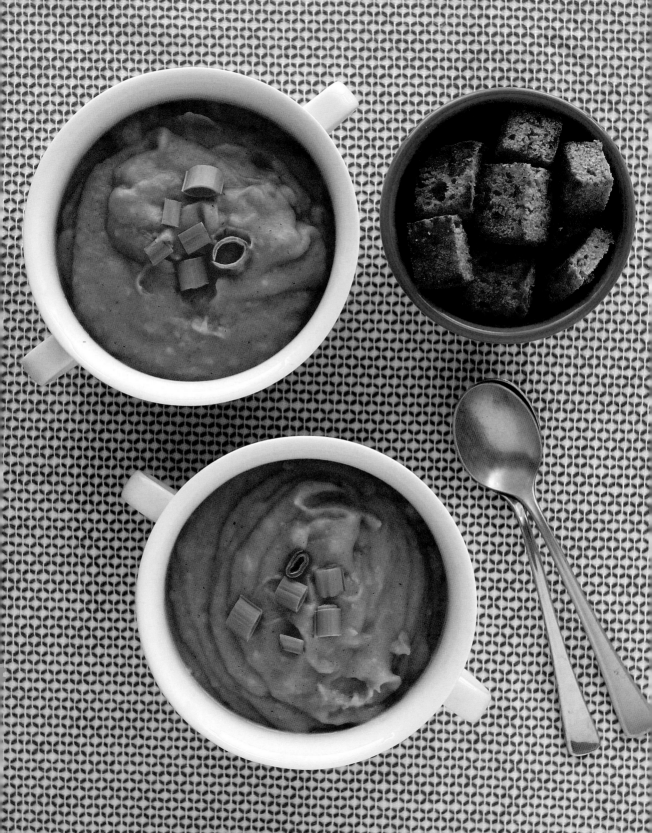

Potato Leek Soup

Potato soup can be made thick and creamy, even without traditional cream, by adding non-dairy milk. This is the soup to make mid to late summer, when both leeks and potatoes are abundant. Luckily, it freezes well, allowing you to save some for a chilly winter night.

1 tablespoon olive oil

3 leeks, washed well and sliced, white and medium-green sections only

8 medium white or yellow potatoes, peeled and diced

Cold water to cover

1 teaspoon salt

½ teaspoon ground black pepper

1 cup (240 ml) Hemp Milk (page 31) or non-dairy milk of choice

1. Heat the olive oil in a large pot over medium heat. Add the leeks and cook until softened, about 8 to 10 minutes.

2. Add the potatoes to the pot with just enough water to cover them. Bring the pot to a low boil, then turn the heat to low. Simmer, uncovered, until the potatoes are tender, about 30 to 45 minutes.

3. When the potatoes are fall-apart tender, use an immersion blender to blend the soup until it is smooth. (Alternatively, transfer the soup in small batches to a blender or food processor to puree, then return it to the pot.) Don't overprocess the soup; a few chunks of potato are fine.

4. Add the salt, pepper, and milk. Simmer for another 10 minutes, or until you are ready to serve.

TO FREEZE

Let the soup cool completely before transferring it to airtight containers. Freeze for up to 6 months. Thaw in the refrigerator; reheat slowly on the stovetop over medium-low heat. When thawing, the water may separate from the soup; retain all of the liquid and add more non-dairy milk, if needed, to achieve the right consistency.

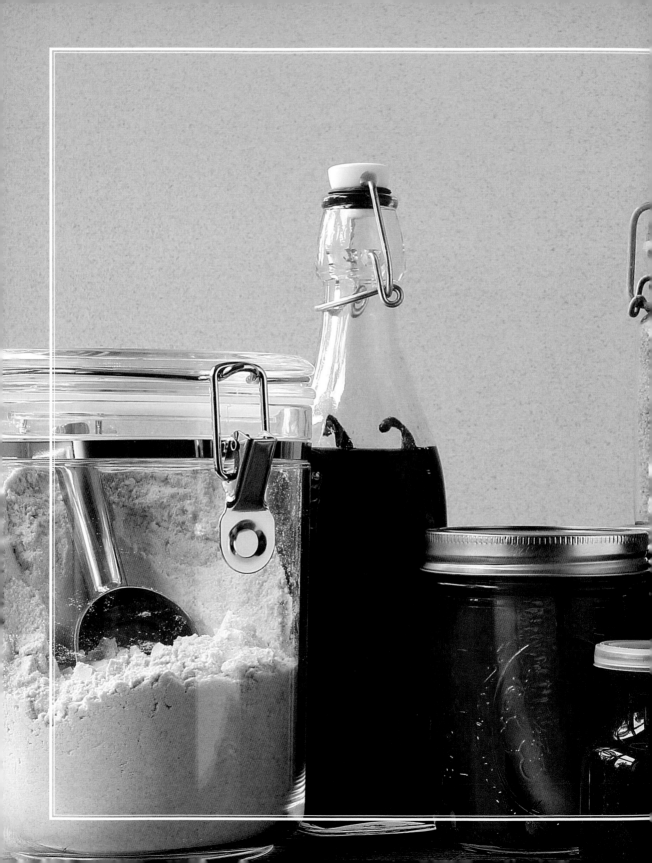

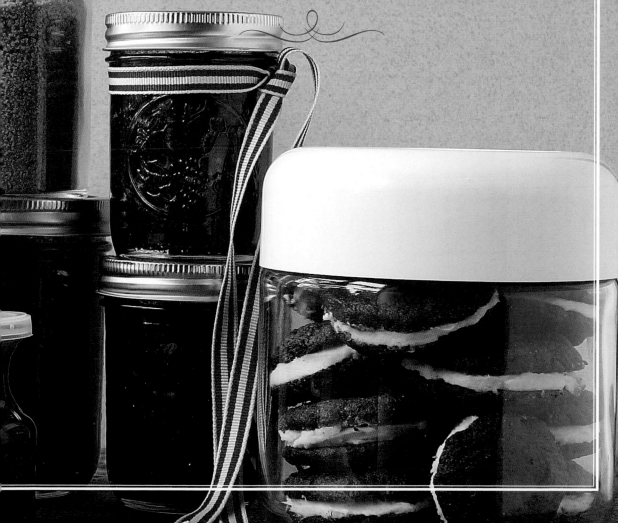

PART 3

SNACKS AND SWEETS

12.

Savory Snacks

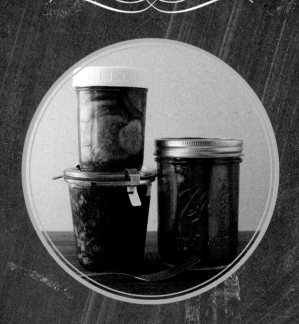

SOFT-BAKED PRETZEL BITES ⌒ DILL PICKLES

POTATO CHIPS ⌒ HUMMUS ⌒ SALSA

Some of us crave sweet snacks and others crave savory snacks. If you fall into the latter category—or you are cooking for someone who does— you will find plenty of allergen-free options here.

If you've never made your own Potato Chips (page 210) or Dill Pickles (page 209), you don't know what you've been missing: homemade versions, void of preservatives, are packed with flavor and allow you to take advantage of fresh, local produce.

Hummus (page 213) and Salsa (page 214) are always best when made fresh—and without the plastic containers.

Many of the recipes in this chapter work equally well as a side dish with other recipes in this book.

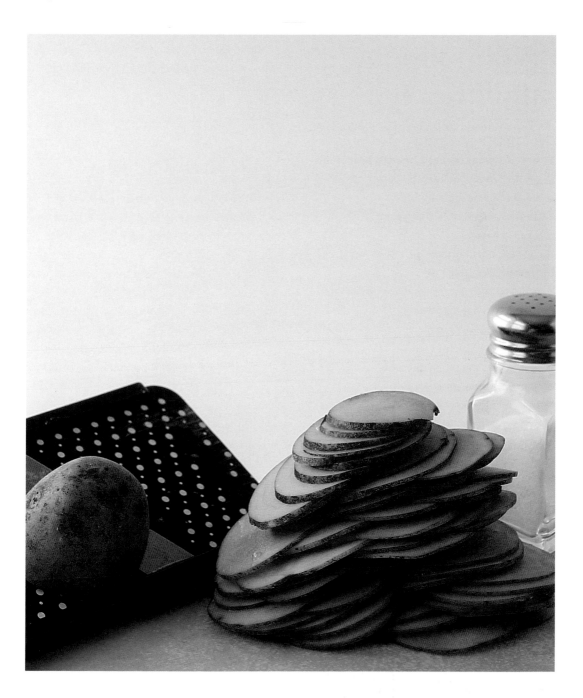

Soft-Baked Pretzel Bites

MAKES ABOUT 40 PRETZEL BITES

*W*alk the streets of New York City and you will find a pretzel vendor on nearly every corner. It's a temptation that some can't resist, but that those of us allergic to wheat must. These easy pretzel bites allow you to indulge at home. Serve them with Honey Mustard Sauce (page 113) for the big game or leave off the salt and dip them in Chocolate Syrup (page 292) for a snack that's savory and sweet.

195 grams (about 1½ cups) Bread Flour Blend (page 23)

30 grams (about ¼ cup) garbanzo bean flour

32 grams (about ¼ cup) tapioca starch

½ teaspoon xanthan gum

2¼ teaspoons quick-rising yeast

½ teaspoon salt

¼ cup (60 ml) sunflower oil

1 Flaxseed Egg (page 42)

½ cup (120 ml) water, plus more for boiling

½ cup (140 g) baking soda

1 to 2 tablespoons coarse sea salt, optional

1. Combine the flours, starch, xanthan gum, yeast, and salt in a medium bowl.

2. In a large bowl, blend together the oil, flaxseed egg, and ½ cup (120 ml) of water using a mixer on medium speed for 30 seconds.

3. Add the dry ingredients and combine them on low speed, then beat for 2 minutes on medium-high speed. Pretzel dough is very thick so that the pretzels hold their shape in the water bath.

4. Let the dough rise in the mixing bowl in a warm, humid spot for 20 minutes.

5. Fill a large pot halfway full with water and the baking soda, and bring to a boil. The water should be at least 3 inches (7.5 cm) deep in the pan.

6. Preheat the oven to 375°F (190°C). Line a large baking sheet with parchment paper.

7. Break off a section of dough. Pat and roll it gently with your fingers to create a log, about ¾ inch (2 cm) thick. Use a flat knife to cut 1¼-inch (3 cm) lengths of dough (or desired length) from the rope. Repeat this step until all of the pretzel bites are shaped.

8. Make sure the water is at a full boil. Use a slotted spoon to carefully place 8 to 10 pretzels at a time into the boiling water. Boil the pretzels for 30 to 45 seconds. Remove the pretzels from the water with the slotted spoon and place them on the baking sheet. Repeat this process until all of the pretzels are boiled.

9. Sprinkle the pretzels with coarse salt, if desired. Leave the salt topping off any you don't plan to eat within 24 hours.

10. Bake for 21 to 23 minutes, until the pretzels are medium brown and have formed a crust.

TO FREEZE

Pretzels you don't plan to eat within 2 days can be frozen in an airtight container for up to 6 months. Thaw them at room temperature; warm at 325°F (165°C) for 5 to 6 minutes, if desired.

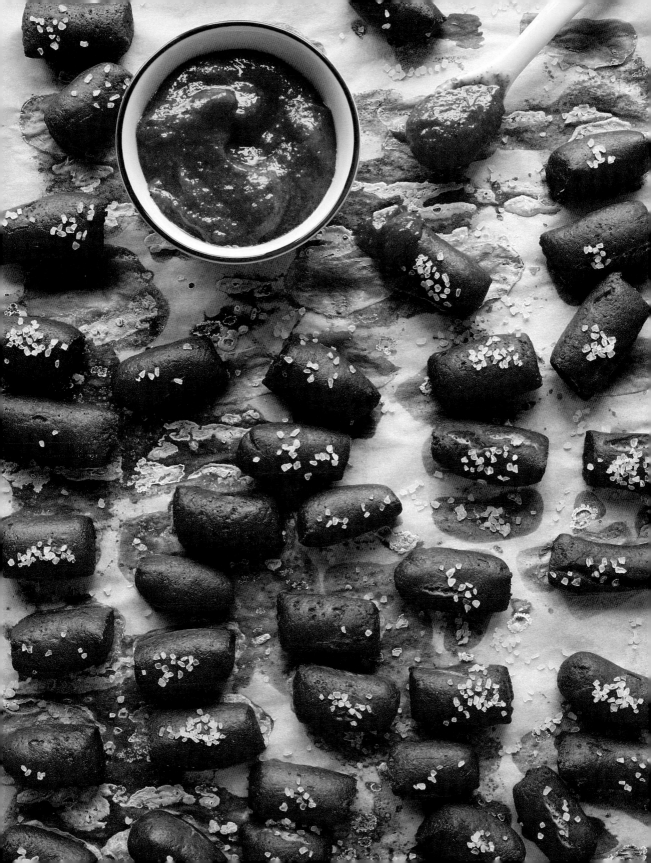

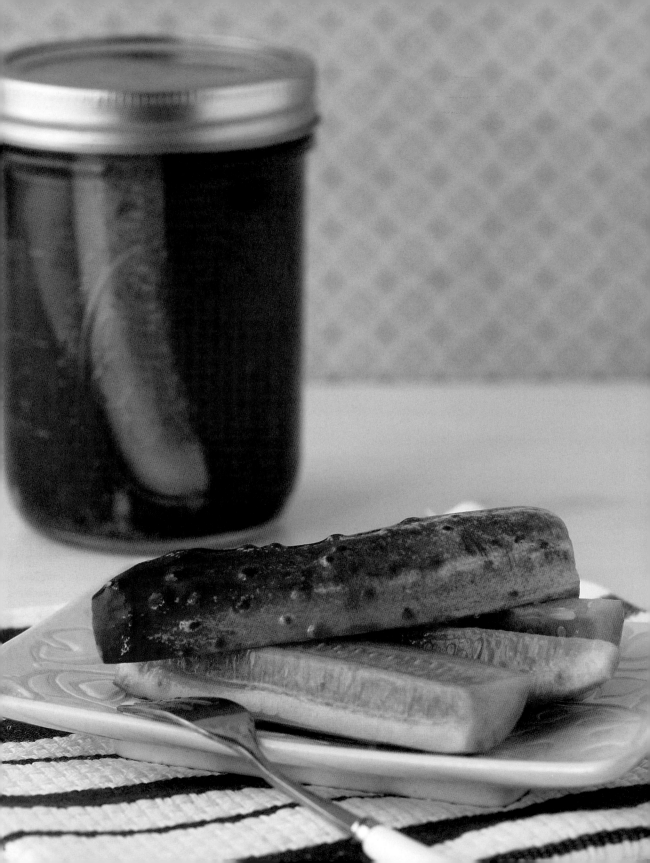

Dill Pickles

MAKES 3 PINTS (1440 ML)
Use three 1-pint (16-ounce/480 ml) jars

*P*ickles can be aged in the refrigerator (these are known as refrigerator pickles) or processed in a water bath and preserved for up to a year. Either way, you will need to sterilize glass jars and use two-part sealing lids. Pickling requires hot-packing with a brine; use vinegar with at least 5 percent acidity (check the label). Use pickling cucumbers to make sure the pickles will snap when you bite into them.

1½ cups (360 ml) apple cider vinegar (5 percent acidity)

1½ cups (360 ml) water

2 tablespoons kosher or pickling salt

4 garlic cloves, chopped

1 teaspoon whole black peppercorns

6 teaspoons chopped fresh dill

7 to 8 medium pickling cucumbers, ends removed, cut into spears

1. Start boiling the jars and preparing the lids, following steps 1 and 2 on page 74 (Steps for Canning). The jars need to boil for a full 10 minutes. You will need to boil the jars even if you aren't canning.

2. Combine the vinegar, water, salt, garlic, peppercorns, and dill in a medium non-reactive saucepan, and bring to a boil.

3. Lower the heat and simmer for 10 minutes, uncovered.

4. Remove the sterilized jars from the canning pot, drain the water from them, and fill them with the cucumbers. Do not overpack the jars; leave at least 1 inch (2.5 cm) of space from the top of the pickles to the top of the jar.

5. Pour the brine over the cucumbers, leaving ½ inch (13 mm) of headspace. Make sure the cucumbers are completely covered with brine. Place the lids on the jars and secure them with rings.

6. If you are making refrigerator pickles, let the filled jars cool and then refrigerate them. Let the pickles age for 1 week before eating (they need time to pickle) and use them within 3 months.

7. Otherwise, you can extend the shelf life of the pickles by processing them in a water bath for 10 minutes (follow steps 6 through 8 on pages 74–75); use them within a year.

Potato Chips

There are two secrets to making crispy potato chips. First, be sure to use russet potatoes. Second, let the sliced potatoes soak for at least an hour in salted water before drying and baking them. Soaking the potatoes removes some of the starchiness, allowing them to crisp up nicely when baked. Use two large (13 by 18-inch/33 by 46 cm) baking sheets for this recipe or make it in two batches.

2 medium-large russet potatoes (one per baking sheet)

Cold water to cover

3 teaspoons salt

1 tablespoon light olive oil

1. Slice the potatoes thinly (¹⁄₁₆ inch/1.5 mm is ideal—see tool tip below).
2. Fill a bowl with cold water and the sliced potatoes. Give them a good swirl in the water and drain. Fill the bowl with clean cold water and 1 teaspoon of salt, and let the potatoes soak for an hour or longer.
3. Drain the potatoes and dry them completely between paper towels. Press hard to remove as much water as you can. (Let the paper towels dry and you can reuse them.)
4. Preheat the oven to 375°F (190°C). Line two large baking sheets with parchment paper.
5. In a clean bowl, toss the potatoes in the olive oil to coat them. Spread the potatoes in a single layer on the baking sheets.
6. Bake the potatoes for 15 minutes. Remove the baking sheets from the oven and sprinkle the chips with the remaining salt, if desired.
7. Reduce the oven heat to 350°F (180°C). Reverse the positions of the baking sheets in the oven for even baking. Bake for 15 minutes.
8. Remove any crispy chips, reverse the positions of the baking sheets in the oven again, and bake for 5 minutes longer, if needed. Repeat this process one more time, if needed. Total baking time is 30 to 40 minutes, depending on the thickness of your chips and your preference for crispiness. Potato Chips are best eaten the day you make them.

Mandoline

You may find a mandoline (sometimes known as mandolin or mandolin slicer) useful to achieve thin slices. I prefer the simplest version of this tool; choose one that has a set slicing option (thin is best) rather than an adjustable blade, and choose a single-bladed version over a model that slices in a V-shape. Safety is of the utmost importance when using any slicer; always use the food holder or cut-resistant gloves to protect your hands.

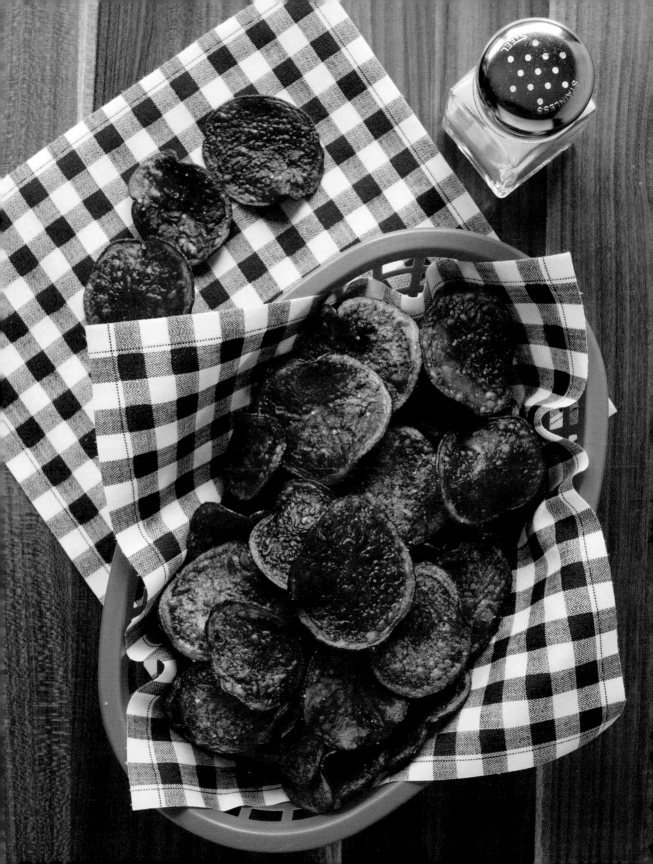

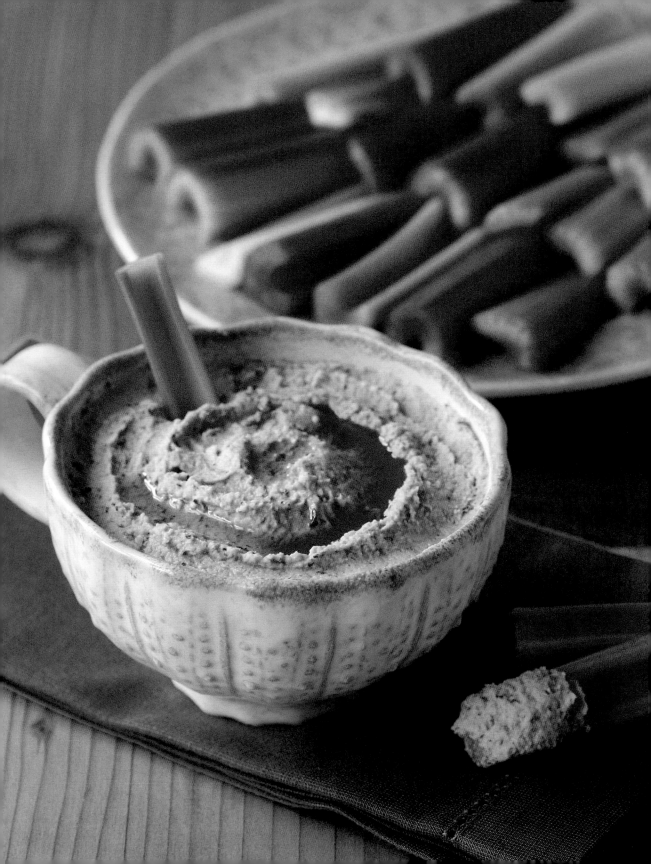

Hummus

Hummus has become a refrigerator staple over the past decade, but families with food allergies often have difficulty finding hummus at the grocery store. Even the plain varieties contain tahini made from sesame—an allergy that is becoming more common, and cross-contamination can be an issue for those allergic to nuts. Leaving out the tahini and making hummus at home is the best solution. Whether you cook your own beans or choose beans from a can, this basic recipe can be enhanced with whatever herbs and vegetables you prefer.

2 cups (425 g) of cooked chickpeas (garbanzo beans), drained (or one 15- to 16-ounce/425 g can chickpeas, drained)

3 tablespoons fresh lemon juice

1 garlic clove

¼ cup (60 ml) olive oil

1 tablespoon chopped fresh parsley

½ teaspoon salt

1. Place the chickpeas, lemon juice, garlic, oil, and parsley in a food processor or high-speed blender and pulse until the ingredients are combined and smooth.
2. Add salt to taste. Cover and refrigerate for up to a week.

TO FREEZE

Freeze in an airtight container for up to 6 months. Thaw in the refrigerator.

Salsa

This fresh salsa, reminiscent of the type you might find at authentic Mexican restaurants, can be made as hot as you like it. Omit the chile pepper for mild, and double it for hot. This recipe is not designed for canning.

2 pounds (908 g) tomatoes, cored (about 5 medium tomatoes)

1 medium chile pepper, seeded and diced

1 small green bell pepper, seeded and diced

1 small onion, peeled and diced

¼ cup (60 ml) roughly chopped fresh cilantro

3 garlic cloves

¼ cup (60 ml) fresh lime juice

½ teaspoon salt

1. Quarter the tomatoes. Remove some of the seeds and drain excess liquid.
2. Dice half of the tomatoes and combine them with the peppers and onions in a large bowl.
3. Place the cilantro and garlic in a food processor or high-speed blender and process on medium-high for 30 seconds. Add the remaining tomatoes and pulse until the mixture is chunky. If the tomatoes are very juicy, you may need to drain some of the liquid.
4. Combine the salsa with the vegetable mixture. Stir in the lime juice. Add salt to taste. Cover leftovers and refrigerate for up to 2 days.

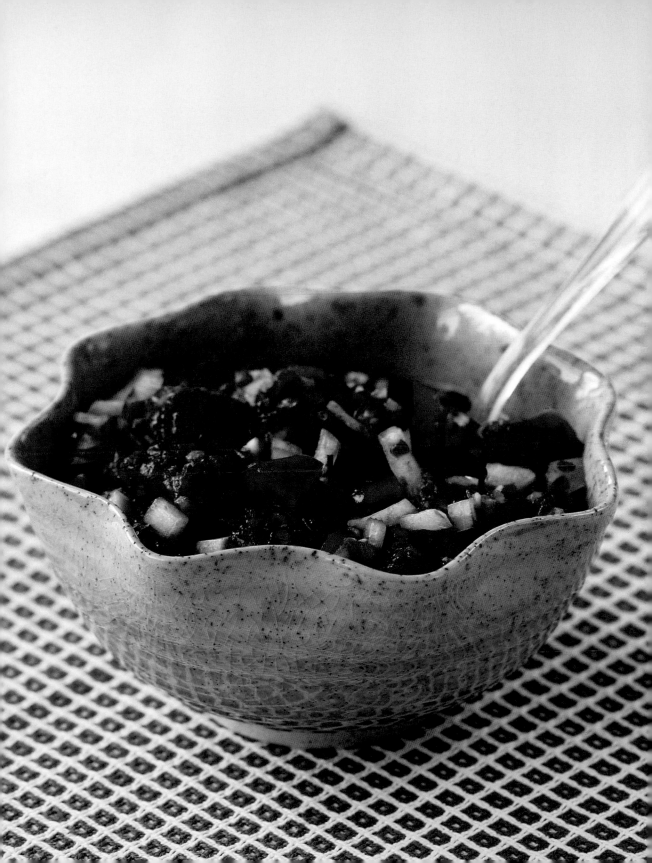

13.

Crackers

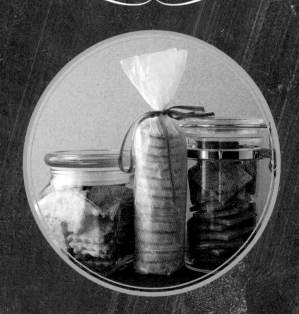

FLAX CRACKERS ⌒ BUTTERY CRACKERS ⌒ SPICY HEMP

CRACKERS ⌒ BUCKWHEAT MAPLE CRACKERS ⌒ PITA CHIPS

Crackers are easy to carry in a purse or bag and can be eaten with your hands. We love them because they are a healthy and versatile snack, usually low in sugar and fat, and they take on flavor from grains, spices, and other ingredients. Instead of searching for a safe package of crackers at the grocery store, make them at home with your choice of ingredients.

Crackers are, in essence, yeast-free, unleavened flatbreads. It may take some practice to get the dough just right, and it will definitely take some muscle to roll the crackers, but once you master the technique you will be able to modify the spices and added ingredients to make just about any cracker you desire. A rolling pin and a heavy hand are needed to roll out crispy crackers; there is no such thing as too thin when it comes to crackers.

None of the crackers in this chapter need a topping to be considered complete. From salty to spicy to slightly sweet, there's a cracker here for everyone.

ABOUT CRACKER DOUGH

Whereas crackers are among the easiest and most satisfying treats to make, getting the hang of cracker dough may take some practice. Most cracker dough is prepared by combining flours with just a small amount of oil and other liquids. The ingredients must be thoroughly mixed, resulting in smooth, dry dough—drier than most dough (the exception being pasta dough).

Don't be afraid to get your hands dirty—they are the tool of choice to blend cracker dough. Properly kneaded cracker dough will be smooth and pliable. The smoother the dough, the easier it will be to roll out; it's nearly impossible to overknead cracker dough.

Because so little moisture is used, it's important to add the wet ingredients slowly. If you are finding it difficult to knead the dough, let it rest (to allow the flour to absorb the liquids) and come back to it after a few minutes. If you need to modify the flour blend used in the cracker recipe, you may need to slightly adjust the liquids. Extra ingredients (such as seeds) should be massaged into the dough (again, with your hands) only after the right texture is achieved.

The balance of wet to dry ingredients is critical with cracker dough, but it's nearly always possible to rescue a cracker project if you add too much or too little liquid. When you are ready to roll out the dough (between two sheets of parchment paper), properly prepared cracker dough will neither stick nor crumble. If the dough sticks to the parchment, scoop it up into a ball, add more flour (1 tablespoon at a time), and massage the flour into the ball until it is smooth. If the dough crumbles, return it to the bowl, add a tiny bit more water, and knead it into a smooth ball.

Rolling pin

Classic wooden rolling pins can be a source of cross-contamination. Purchase a separate rolling pin for use with allergen-free foods, or invest in a nonporous rolling pin.

Preparing Cracker Dough

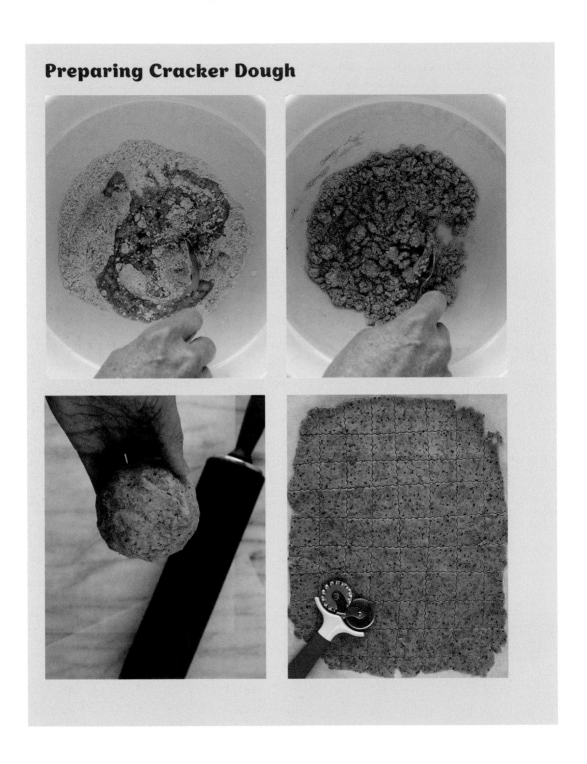

The best method to make crackers is with your hands and a rolling pin (see tool tip on page 219) following these steps:

1. Combine the dry ingredients in a large bowl.

2. Add the oil and other wet ingredients, reserving 1 tablespoon of water. Unless otherwise specified, all ingredients should be at room temperature. Use a spoon to incorporate the wet ingredients, then use your hands to knead them together, working the fat into the dough.

3. Add the remaining water as needed, ½ tablespoon at a time, and continue kneading until the dough is smooth. It should hold together but not be wet. It can be helpful to let the dough rest for a few minutes, come back to it, and work it longer.

4. In rare cases (e.g., if you modified a flour blend) it may be necessary to add more liquid than the recipe suggests; if needed, add up to 1 more tablespoon of water, ½ tablespoon at a time, to achieve the right consistency.

5. Roll the dough out between two sheets of parchment paper. Use additional flour, if needed, to prevent the dough from sticking to the parchment. Roll from the center to the edges. The thinner you roll the dough the crispier the crackers will be and the less time it will take for them to bake. When you think you have rolled the crackers as thinly as possible, roll one more time (except where directed to roll to a specific thickness, as in Buttery Crackers, page 224).

From here, the dough can be scored, cut into shapes, or baked as a sheet, according to the recipe.

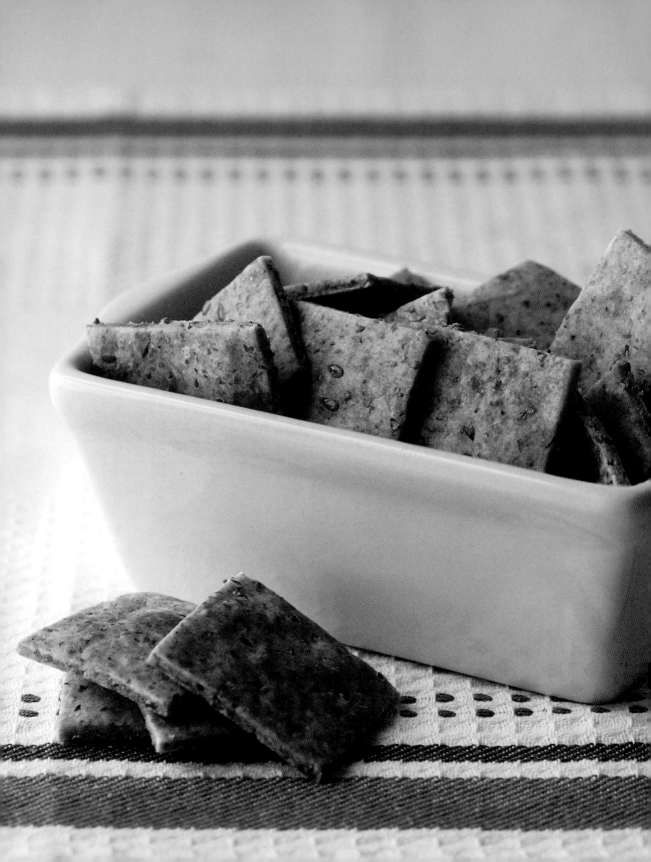

Flax Crackers

This cracker contains a healthy dose of flaxseeds, giving it great flavor as well as fiber and essential fatty acids. Its texture makes for a great snack and successful dipping, as it mimics traditional wheat thins—without the wheat, of course.

130 grams (about 1 cup) Bread Flour Blend (page 23)

½ teaspoon xanthan gum

2 tablespoons flaxseed meal

¼ teaspoon salt

2 tablespoons grapeseed oil

1 tablespoon agave nectar

3 to 4 tablespoons water

1. Preheat the oven to 400°F (200°C).
2. Combine the flour, xanthan gum, 1 tablespoon flaxseed meal, and salt in a large mixing bowl.
3. Add the oil, agave nectar, and 3 tablespoons of water. Use a spoon to combine the ingredients, then use your hands to knead the liquids into the dough. Add up to 1 tablespoon of additional water as needed, ½ tablespoon at a time, until the dough is smooth. (See Preparing Cracker Dough on page 220.)
4. Sprinkle the remaining flaxseed meal on a large piece of parchment paper. Place the dough on top of the flaxseed meal and roll it into a ball, coating all sides with flaxseed meal.
5. Place a second piece of parchment paper on top of the dough. Use a rolling pin to roll the dough between the sheets of parchment, working to within ½ inch (13 mm) of the edges. Peel back the top layer of parchment and move the bottom layer of parchment (with the dough) to the baking sheet.
6. Use a sharp knife or pizza cutter to score the crackers. Leave them connected.
7. Bake for 9 to 11 minutes, until lightly browned. Let the crackers cool before breaking them apart. Store them in an airtight container at room temperature for up to 3 days.

TO FREEZE

Crackers that won't be eaten within 2 to 3 days can be frozen in airtight containers for up to 6 months; thaw them at room temperature. Cracker dough (prepared through step 3) can be wrapped tightly in plastic and frozen for up to 6 months; thaw the dough in the refrigerator and then let it sit at room temperature for an hour before continuing with step 4.

Buttery Crackers

Instead of traditional Ritz crackers, try substituting these crackers. They are flaky, buttery (without the dairy), and salty with just a hint of sweet. Serve them with your favorite soup, or add a layer of Sunflower Seed Butter (page 77) to build cracker sandwiches (see variation).

98 grams (about ¾ cup) Bread Flour Blend (page 23)

32 grams (about ¼ cup) Pastry Flour Blend (page 24)

½ teaspoon xanthan gum

2 teaspoons organic cane sugar

1 teaspoon baking powder

¾ teaspoon salt

2 tablespoons coconut oil, melted

3 to 4 tablespoons water

1. Preheat the oven to 375°F (190°C). Line a large baking sheet with parchment paper.
2. Combine the flours, xanthan gum, sugar, baking powder, and ½ teaspoon salt in a large mixing bowl.
3. Add the oil and 3 tablespoons of water. Use a spoon to combine the ingredients, then use your hands to knead the liquids into the dough. Add up to 1 tablespoon of additional water as needed, ½ tablespoon at a time, until the dough is smooth. (See Preparing Cracker Dough on page 220.)
4. Place the dough between two sheets of parchment paper and roll to ⅛ inch (3 mm) thick. Remove the top sheet of parchment. Use a small cookie cutter or biscuit cutter to create crackers about 1¼ inches (3 cm) round.
5. Remove excess dough and transfer the formed crackers to the prepared baking sheet, with space in between. Roll out the remaining dough, cut crackers, and transfer them to the baking sheet, until all of the dough is used.
6. Use a fork to poke tiny holes into the crackers. Sprinkle the tops of the crackers with the remaining salt, if desired.
7. Bake for 9 to 10 minutes, until the tops are just golden. Store them in an airtight container at room temperature for up to 3 days.

VARIATION

To make Sunflower Butter Filled Crackers, spread ¾ teaspoon of Sunflower Seed Butter (page 77) between two Buttery Crackers. (This combination is pictured on page 76.)

TO SUBSTITUTE

To make a coconut-free version, substitute another shortening (see page 7).

TO FREEZE

Crackers that won't be eaten within 2 to 3 days can be frozen in an airtight container for up to 6 months; bring them to room temperature before serving. Cracker dough (prepared through step 3) can be wrapped tightly in plastic and frozen for up to 6 months; thaw the dough in the refrigerator and then let it sit at room temperature for an hour before rolling.

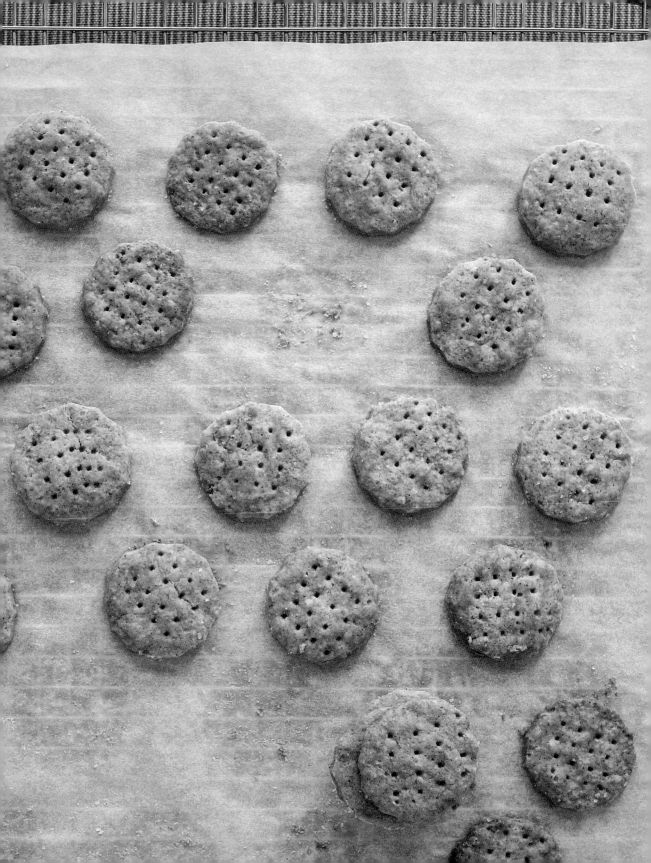

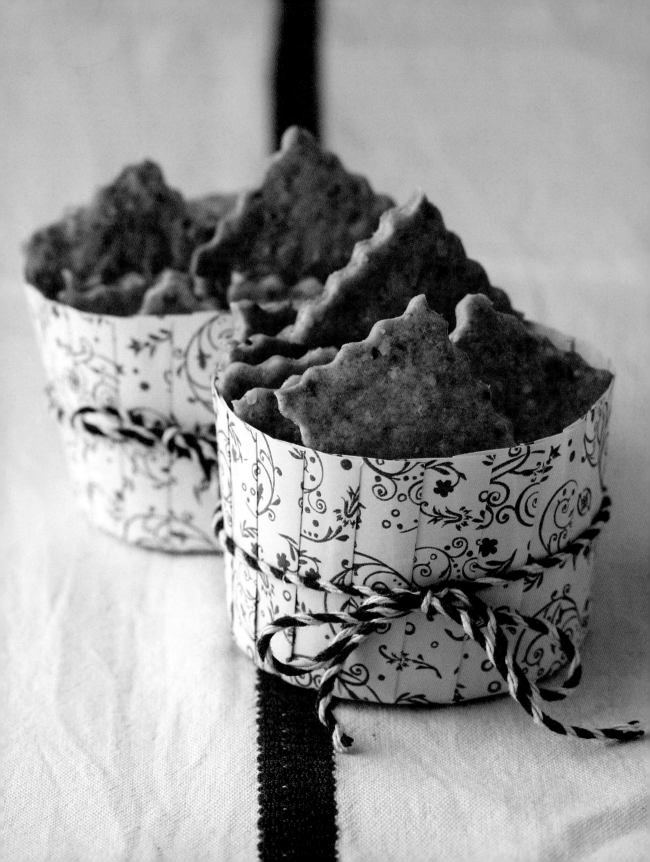

Spicy Hemp Crackers

||||||||||||||||||||||||||||||||||||||||||||||||||||||||||||||||||||||||||||||||||||||||||||||||||||||||||||||||||||||||||||||||||||||||||||||||||||||||||||||||||||||||||||

T his cracker is just right for parties or for carrying in your bag for an anytime pick-me-up. Although they contain no dairy, they do have a slightly cheesy taste provided by shelled hemp seeds and spices. The flavor is built right in!

98 grams (about ¾ cup) Pastry Flour Blend (page 24)

30 grams (about ¼ cup) millet flour

½ teaspoon xanthan gum

¼ cup (40 g) shelled hemp seeds

½ teaspoon salt

¼ teaspoon ground black pepper

¼ teaspoon paprika

2 tablespoons light olive oil

3 to 4 tablespoons water

1. Preheat the oven to 400°F (200°C).
2. Combine the flours, xanthan gum, hemp seeds, salt, pepper, and paprika in a large mixing bowl.
3. Add the oil and 3 tablespoons of water. Use a spoon to combine the ingredients, then use your hands to knead the liquids into the dough. Add up to 1 tablespoon of additional water as needed, ½ tablespoon at a time, until the dough is smooth. (See Preparing Cracker Dough on page 220.)
4. Place the dough between two sheets of parchment paper. Use a rolling pin to roll the dough thinly, working to within 1 inch (2.5 cm) of the edges. Use additional flour, if needed, to avoid sticking.
5. Peel back the top layer of parchment and move the bottom layer of parchment (with the dough) to the baking sheet. Use a sharp knife or cutter to score the crackers. Leave them connected.
6. Bake for 12 to 14 minutes, until lightly browned. Let the crackers cool before breaking them apart. Store them in an airtight container at room temperature for up to 3 days.

TO FREEZE

Crackers that won't be eaten within 2 to 3 days can be frozen in an airtight container for up to 6 months; bring them to room temperature before serving. Cracker dough (prepared through step 3) can be wrapped tightly in plastic and frozen for up to 6 months; thaw the dough in the refrigerator and then let it sit at room tempera-ture for an hour before rolling.

VARIATION

For a cheesier cracker, work ¼ cup (28 g) Daiya Cheddar Style Shreds (chopped into ¼-inch/6.5 mm pieces) into the dough after step 3 and prior to rolling the crackers.

Buckwheat Maple Crackers   MAKES ABOUT 50 CRACKERS

These crackers remind me of a childhood trip to New Hampshire, where I was introduced to decadent candies made with pure maple sugar. Here, I combine that same melt-in-your-mouth goodness with buckwheat. Despite its name, buckwheat is not related to wheat; ground from seeds (known as groats), buckwheat flour is a great source of fiber and protein. These crackers are prepared similar to cookies.

128 grams (about 1 cup) Basic Flour Blend (page 23)

80 grams (about ½ cup) buckwheat flour

¼ teaspoon xanthan gum

¼ cup (42 g) maple sugar

½ teaspoon salt

8 tablespoons shortening (see page 7), cold

¼ cup (60 ml) pure maple syrup, cold

Up to 2 tablespoons cold water, as needed

1. Combine the flours, xanthan gum, maple sugar, and salt in a large mixing bowl.
2. Cut the shortening into tablespoon-sized pieces and lay them on top of the flour.
3. Use a pastry cutter or pastry fork to work the shortening into the flour. After 3 to 4 minutes of cutting the mixture will be crumbly.
4. Add the maple syrup and work it into the dough with the pastry cutter. Add up to 2 tablespoons of cold water as needed, ½ tablespoon at a time, until the dough forms. (See Preparing Cookie Dough on page 236.)
5. Work the dough into a flattened rectangle. Wrap it in plastic and refrigerate for at least an hour. Dough can be refrigerated for up to 2 weeks.
6. When you are ready to bake the crackers, preheat the oven to 375°F (190°C).
7. Place the dough between two sheets of parchment paper. Use a rolling pin to roll the dough to within 1 inch (2.5 cm) of the edges of the parchment.
8. Peel back the top layer of parchment and move the bottom layer of parchment (with the dough) to the baking sheet. If pieces of dough fall off while peeling, simply stick them back together with your fingers.
9. Use a sharp knife or pizza cutter to score the crackers. Leave them connected.
10. Bake for 15 to 16 minutes, until the crackers are lightly browned. Let the crackers cool before breaking them apart. Store them at room temperature for up to 3 days.

TO FREEZE

Crackers that won't be eaten within 2 to 3 days can be frozen in an airtight container for up to 6 months; bring them to room temperature before serving. Cracker dough (prepared through step 5) can be frozen for up to 6 months; thaw it in the refrigerator before continuing with step 6.

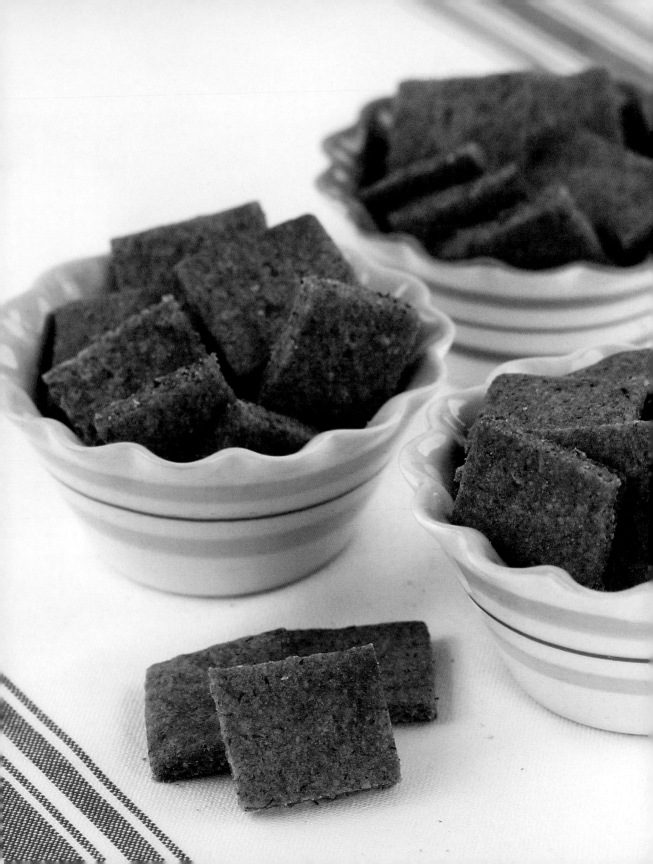

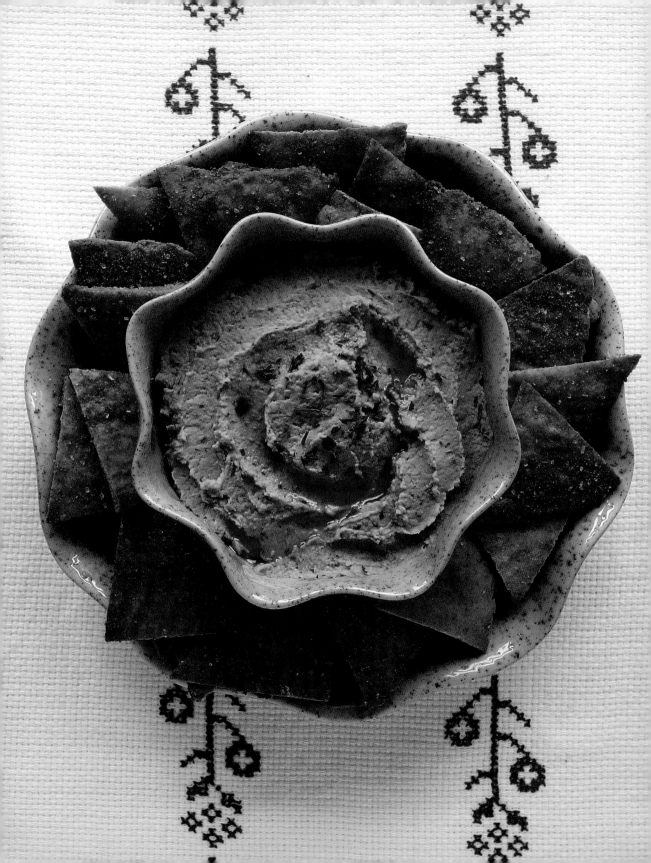

Pita Chips

Pita Chips are a cross between a chip and a cracker. They work equally well alongside a sandwich or with your favorite dip. Use any combination of oils and seasoning that you prefer to vary the flavor of these chips. These chips are best eaten within 2 days.

Four 5-inch (13 cm) Flatbreads (page 68)
1½ tablespoons light olive oil
¼ teaspoon salt
1 teaspoon cumin
1 teaspoon garlic powder

1. Cut each flatbread in half and gently score the centers to create 2 sides (as if you were making a pita pocket). Cut each half into 3 triangles, then separate the two sides of each triangle to create two chips. Each flatbread will yield 12 chips.

2. Line a large baking sheet with parchment paper. Preheat the oven to 375°F (190°C).

3. Place the chips on the baking sheet, without overlap. Brush each chip on both sides with oil.

4. Mix the salt, cumin, and garlic powder together and sprinkle the mixture on top of the chips.

5. Bake for 8 minutes. Remove any thinner chips that are already browned and crispy. Bake for 2 minutes longer and remove any crispy chips. If needed, bake the remaining chips for another 2 minutes.

6. Let the chips cool before serving. Store them in an airtight container at room temperature for 2 days.

14.

Cookies

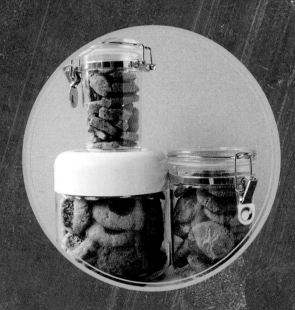

CHOCOLATE CHIP COOKIES ❧ CHOCOLATE SANDWICH COOKIES

SNICKERDOODLES ❧ FIG-FILLED COOKIES

STRAWBERRY THUMBPRINTS ❧ ANIMAL CRACKERS

All parents dream of greeting their smiling children with a plate of freshly baked cookies as they arrive home after school. Yes, it's just a dream. In reality, the kids aren't always smiling and most of us don't have the luxury of being able to bake in the middle of the afternoon. Instead, we rely on store-bought snacks, but a box of store-bought cookies that is safe for your child is likely expensive and may contain just a handful of cookies.

This chapter offers easy recipes for your favorite cookies, including Chocolate Chip Cookies (page 238), Snickerdoodles (page 245), and Thumbprints (page 249). There are cookies for kids of all ages (and most can be made with help from the kids). If you prepare the dough in advance and keep some cookie dough rolls in the refrigerator, you will be able to slice up just a few cookies (or a whole batch) and pop them into the oven when you need them—after school, for a playdate, or to treat yourself!

ABOUT COOKIE DOUGH

Some of the cookies (such as Chocolate Chip Cookies, page 238) in this chapter are made by hand using a method called cutting, in which chilled shortening is worked into the dough. Small chunks of shortening will remain whole while most of the shortening will coat the flour and sugar. When the cookie dough forms you will be able to roll it into a log. Cookie dough rolls must be chilled for at least an hour (to allow the shortening to harden) before slicing cookies, but the dough will last in the refrigerator for up to 2 weeks and even longer in the freezer.

Your choice of shortening (see page 7) will affect how much liquid you need to add to the dough and how long you need to refrigerate before baking. If you use a modified flour blend, the amount of liquid you need to add to the dough may also vary. The wet ingredients should be added slowly to achieve just the right texture—not too dry yet not too sticky.

Another technique used to prepare some cookies (such as Snickerdoodles, page 245) is called creaming. For these recipes you must use an electric mixer—its speed is required to cream properly. When creaming you will use the shortening at room temperature (unless you need to select a spread—see page 7—in which case you should use it just slightly softened).

Use your mixer to cream together the sugar and shortening on medium speed for about 5 minutes. During this time the sugar will be coated with fat to form a mixture that is both fluffy and grainy; you should be able to feel the graininess when you scrape down the bowl of the mixer. Both the speed of the mixer and the length of time you mix are critical to achieving the right texture. A crystal (not liquid) form of sugar must be used for creaming. Follow the recipe to determine whether cookies that are prepared using creaming should be chilled prior to baking.

Pastry cutter

A pastry cutter (sometimes called a pastry blender, dough blender, or dough cutter) is the preferred tool to cut shortening into flour when making some cookies or pie crusts. This simple, inexpensive tool has blades on the bottom to work the shortening into the dough and a sturdy handle on top. Alternatives include a pastry fork (a large fork with wide prongs) or your hands.

Preparing Cookie Dough

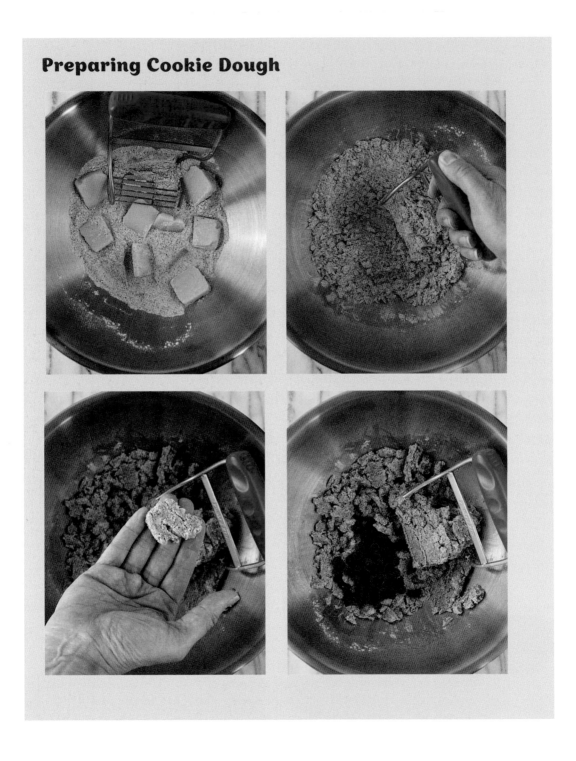

Some cookies are made without a stand mixer or whisk. Instead, a hands-on method called cutting (or rubbing) is used. After combining the dry ingredients in a large bowl, follow these steps:

1. Cut the shortening into tablespoon-sized pieces and lay them on top of the dry ingredients. You will achieve the best results if you select a shortening that remains solid at room temperature (see page 7 to learn about shortening options).

2. Use a pastry cutter (see tool tip on page 235) to work the shortening into the flour. Unlike batters or cracker dough (where the fat is completely incorporated into the mix), some of the shortening in cookie dough will remain in tiny pieces. Continue working the shortening into the flour until the mixture is crumbly. This step usually takes 3 to 4 minutes (less time if a spread is used in place of shortening, see page 7). Scrape the dough off the blades of the cutter, as needed.

3. Add the wet ingredients and cut them into the dough. If needed, add more liquid (by ½ tablespoon), until the dough is formed. The dough should stick together, but it shouldn't be wet. The texture of properly prepared cookie dough should be similar to the damp sand you would use to make a sand-castle. If the dough feels too crumbly, add more liquid. When you can see "sheets" of dough coming off the pastry cutter, the dough is complete.

From here, the dough can be refrigerated, rolled, formed, and/or filled, according to the recipe.

Chocolate Chip Cookies

MAKES ABOUT 28 COOKIES

||||||||||||||||||||||||||||||||||||||||||||||||||||||||||||||||||||||||||||||||||||||||||||||||||||||||||||||||||||||||||||||||||||||||||||||||||

Chocolate Chip Cookies are a classic and always my first choice. They are easy to pack in a lunch bag and a favorite at class parties and fund-raisers. If you try just one cookie recipe, this is the one to choose. Bake just a few cookies at a time, make the entire batch, or save some of the dough to make Chocolate Chip Cookie Dough Muffins (page 127)—it's up to you.

96 grams (about ¾ cup) Pastry Flour Blend (page 24)

80 grams (about ½ cup) buckwheat flour

¼ teaspoon xanthan gum

½ cup (110 g) organic cane sugar

1½ teaspoons baking powder

½ teaspoon salt

8 tablespoons shortening (see page 7), cold

2 tablespoons Applesauce (page 45)

1 teaspoon Vanilla Extract (page 288)

Up to 1 tablespoon cold water (as needed)

½ cup (120 g) mini or regular-sized chocolate chips

1. Combine the flours, xanthan gum, sugar, baking powder, and salt in a large mixing bowl.
2. Cut the shortening into tablespoon-sized pieces and lay them on top of the flour. Use a pastry cutter, a pastry fork, or your hands to work the shortening into the flour. Continue working for 3 to 4 minutes, until a crumbly mixture forms.
3. Add the applesauce and vanilla and work the liquids into the dough. Add up to 1 tablespoon of cold water as needed, ½ tablespoon at a time, until the dough forms. (See Preparing Cookie Dough on page 236.)
4. Add the chocolate chips and work them into the dough with your hands.

5. Separate the dough into two sections and roll each section into a cylinder, about 1½ inches (4 cm) thick and 6 inches (15 cm) long. Wrap the rolls tightly in plastic and refrigerate for at least an hour. Cookie dough rolls can be refrigerated for up to 2 weeks.
6. When you are ready to bake the cookies, preheat the oven to 350°F (180°C). Line two large baking sheets with parchment paper.
7. Slice the cookies from the roll, about ⅜ inch (10 mm) thick. Place the cookies on the baking sheets, with space in between. If the dough breaks apart, simply stick it back together.
8. Bake each sheet of cookies separately, in the center of the oven, for 11 to 13 minutes. Let the cookies cool on the baking sheet for 5 minutes, then transfer them to a cooling rack. Store them in an airtight container at room temperature for up to 3 days.

TO FREEZE

Baked cookies can be frozen in an airtight container for up to 3 months; thaw them at room temperature. Freeze cookie dough rolls (prepared through step 5) for up to 6 months; thaw the dough in the refrigerator before slicing and baking.

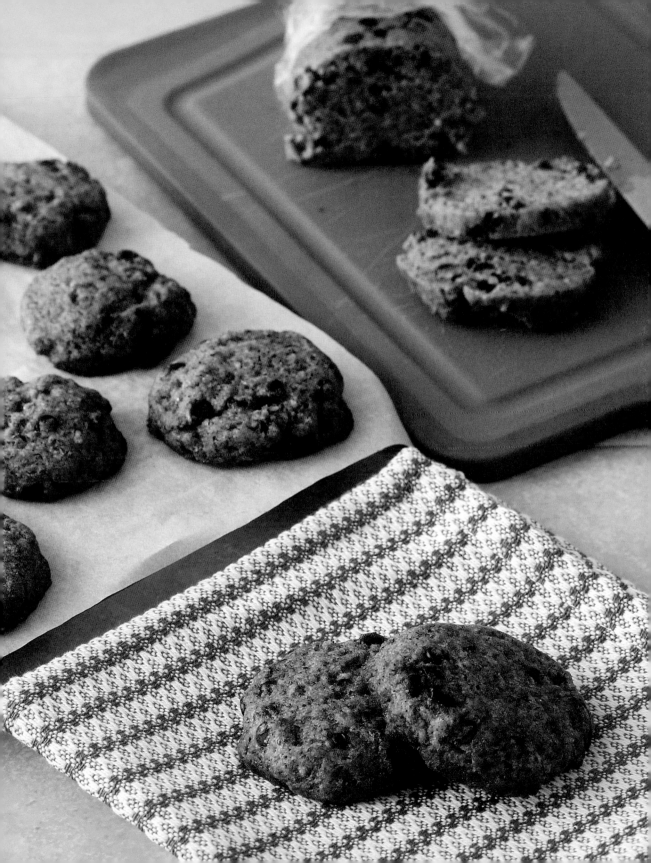

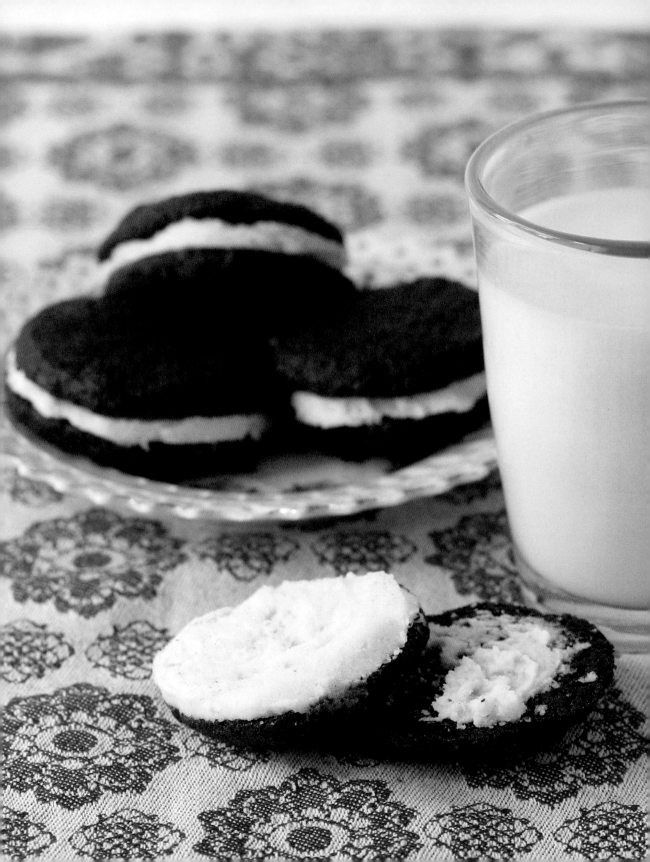

Chocolate Sandwich Cookies

**MAKES ABOUT 14 SANDWICH COOKIES
or 28 wafer cookies**

You won't find any wheat in this chocolate sandwich cookie, yet it tastes just as good as the traditional kind. Dunk it in your favorite non-dairy milk. The chocolate cookie dough can be prepared as wafers without the sugary filling, or with ½ cup of chocolate chips mixed in for a double chocolate treat.

FOR THE CHOCOLATE COOKIE DOUGH

96 grams (about ¾ cup) Pastry Flour Blend (page 24)

80 grams (about ½ cup) buckwheat flour

¼ teaspoon xanthan gum

½ cup (52 g) natural unsweetened cocoa powder

½ cup (110 g) organic cane sugar

1½ teaspoons baking powder

½ teaspoon salt

12 tablespoons shortening (see page 7), cold

2 tablespoons Applesauce (page 45)

1 teaspoon Vanilla Extract (page 288)

Up to 2 tablespoons cold water (as needed)

FOR THE FILLING

1 cup (265 g) Vanilla Frosting (page 294)

To make the cookies

1. Combine the flours, xanthan gum, cocoa powder, sugar, baking powder, and salt in a large mixing bowl.
2. Cut the shortening into tablespoon-sized pieces and lay them on top of the flour. Use a pastry cutter, a pastry fork, or your hands to work the shortening into the flour. Continue working for 3 to 4 minutes, until a crumbly mixture forms.
3. Add the applesauce and vanilla and work the liquids into the dough. Add up to 2 tablespoons of cold water as needed, ½ tablespoon at a time, until the dough forms. (See Preparing Cookie Dough on page 236.)
4. Separate the dough into two sections and roll each into a cylinder about 1½ inches (4 cm) thick and 6 inches (15 cm) long. Wrap the rolls tightly in plastic and refrigerate for at least an hour. Cookie dough rolls can be refrigerated for up to 2 weeks.
5. When you are ready to bake the cookies, preheat the oven to 350°F (180°C). Line two large baking sheets with parchment paper.
6. Slice the cookies from the roll, about ⅜ inch (10 mm) thick. Place the cookies on the baking sheets with space in between. If the dough breaks apart, simply stick it back together.
7. Bake each sheet of cookies separately, in the center of the oven, for 11 to 13 minutes. Let the cookies cool on the baking sheet for 5 minutes, then move them to a cooling rack. Store unfilled cookies in an airtight container at room temperature for up to 3 days.

(recipe continues)

To fill the cookie sandwiches

8. When completely cooled, arrange the cookies in pairs, aligning like sizes and shapes.

9. Spread a layer of frosting on the flat side of the first cookie in each pair; use about 1 tablespoon of frosting per cookie. Lay the second cookie on top, flat side down, and gently press them together. Filled cookies are best eaten the day they are made.

TO FREEZE

Unfilled, baked cookies can be frozen in an airtight container for up to 3 months; thaw them at room temperature. Freeze cookie dough rolls (prepared through step 4) for up to 6 months; thaw the dough in the refrigerator before slicing, baking, cooling, and filling.

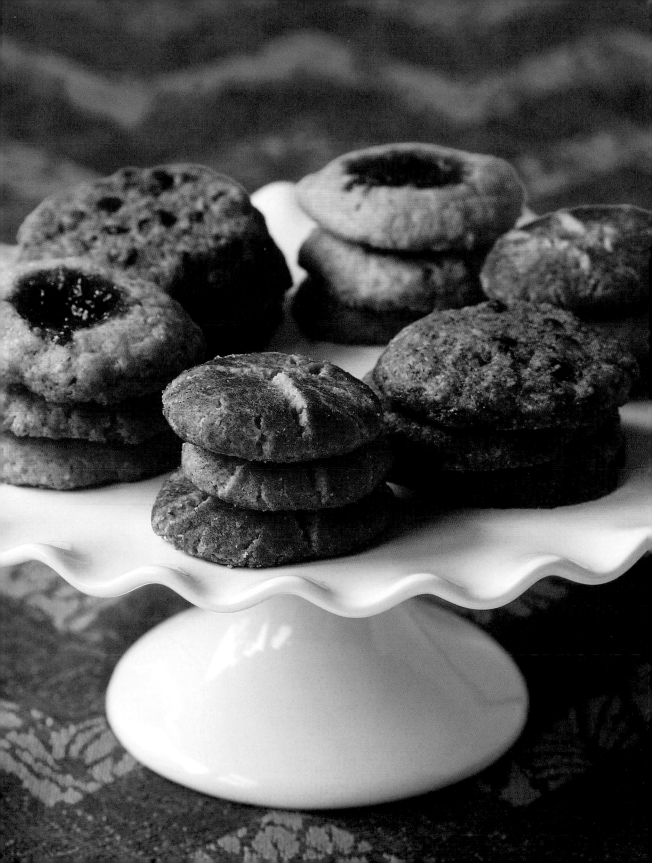

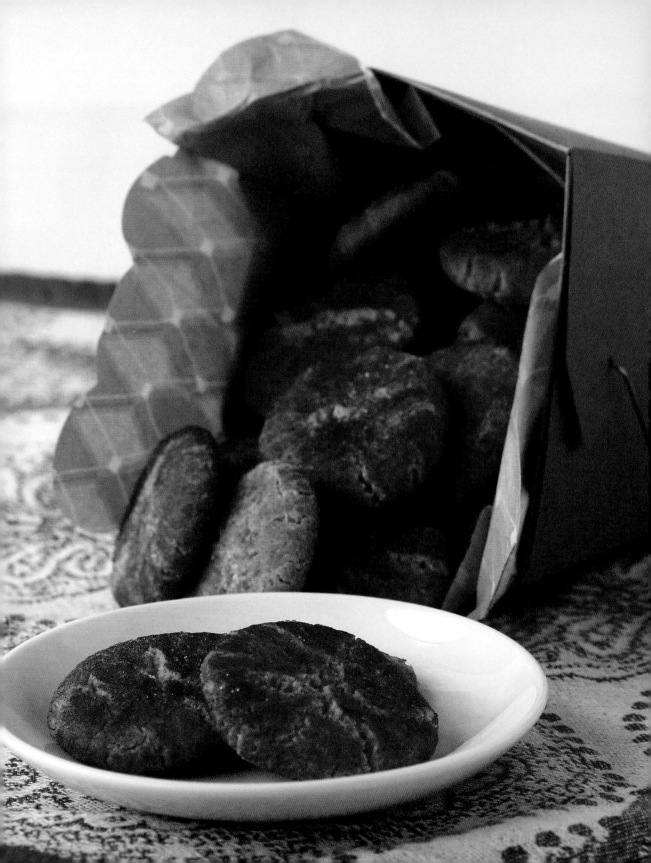

Snickerdoodles

Snickerdoodles may be the easiest cookies on the planet to make, and yet they can be finicky. The trick is to start with a fluffy batter by creaming together the shortening and a crystal form of sugar. The result is a sugary coated cookie with just the right amount of crunch. Yes, the sugar is essential!

This recipe is not suitable for making refrigerator or freezer dough rolls.

195 grams (about 1½ cups) Pastry Flour Blend (page 24)

½ teaspoon xanthan gum

2 teaspoons baking powder

¼ teaspoon salt

¼ teaspoon ground cinnamon

¼ cup (36 g) organic light brown sugar

8 tablespoons shortening (see page 7), softened

½ cup (110 g) organic cane sugar

1 teaspoon Vanilla Extract (page 288)

2 tablespoons apple cider vinegar

3 tablespoons Cinnamon Sugar (page 286)

1. Preheat the oven to 350°F (180°C). Line two large baking sheets with parchment paper.
2. Combine the flour, xanthan gum, baking powder, salt, cinnamon, and brown sugar in a medium bowl.
3. In a separate large bowl, cream together the shortening and cane sugar using a mixer on medium speed for 5 minutes, scraping down the sides of the bowl as needed. The mixture will be light and fluffy.
4. Add the vanilla and vinegar and mix for 30 seconds. Add in the dry ingredients and blend on medium speed, about 2 minutes, until the dough clusters in the center of the mixing bowl.
5. Use your hands to shape the dough into balls about 1¼ inches (3 cm) round.
6. Place the cinnamon sugar in a small shallow bowl. Roll the cookies in the sugar to coat them on all sides. Place the cookies on the baking sheets with space in between and flatten them just slightly.
7. Bake each sheet of cookies separately, in the center of the oven, for 10 minutes. Let the cookies cool on the baking sheet for 5 minutes, then transfer them to a cooling rack. Store them in an airtight container at room temperature for up to 3 days.

TO FREEZE

Baked cookies can be frozen in an airtight container for up to 3 months. Thaw cookies at room temperature before serving.

Fig-Filled Cookies

A cookie filled with jam—now that's decadent. This allergen-free version of a certain popular cookie uses Figgy Pear Jam (page 85) as the filling, but feel free to choose another jam to fill yours.

98 grams (about ¾ cup) Pastry Flour Blend (page 24)

80 grams (about ½ cup) buckwheat flour

½ teaspoon xanthan gum

¼ cup (55 g) organic cane sugar

¼ teaspoon salt

6 tablespoons shortening (see page 7), cold

1 tablespoon apple cider vinegar

½ teaspoon Vanilla Extract (page 288)

3 tablespoons coconut milk beverage or non-dairy milk of choice

½ cup (140 g) Figgy Pear Jam (page 85)

1. Combine the flours, xanthan gum, sugar, and salt in a large mixing bowl.
2. Cut the shortening into tablespoon-sized pieces and lay them on top of the flour. Use a pastry cutter, a pastry fork, or your hands to work the shortening into the flour. Continue working for 3 to 4 minutes, until a crumbly mixture forms.
3. Add the vinegar, vanilla, and milk. Work the liquids into the dough. (See Preparing Cookie Dough on page 236.)
4. Separate the dough into two equal sections. Roll each section between two pieces of parchment paper to create two sheets of dough about 4 inches (10 cm) wide, 8 inches (20 cm) long, and ¼ inch (6.5 mm) thick in the center, with the edges tapering to a thinner ⅛ inch (3 mm) thick.
5. Spread half of the jam down the center of one dough sheet. Fold one side of the dough over the jam, then fold the second side over the first to create a log. Gently flip the log over so that the folded side is on the bottom; repair any cracks with a small amount of water and your fingers. Repeat this process with the second sheet and the remaining jam. Refrigerate the filled logs for at least an hour. (If you plan to refrigerate longer than an hour, wrap the logs in plastic.)
6. When you are ready to bake the cookies, preheat the oven to 350°F (180°C). Line a large baking sheet with parchment paper.
7. Slice each log into 8 cookies, about 1 inch (2.5 cm) long. Place the cookies on the baking sheet, with space in between.
8. Bake for 14 to 16 minutes, until lightly browned. Let the cookies cool on the baking sheet for 5 minutes, then transfer them to a cooling rack. Store them in an airtight container at room temperature for up to 2 days.

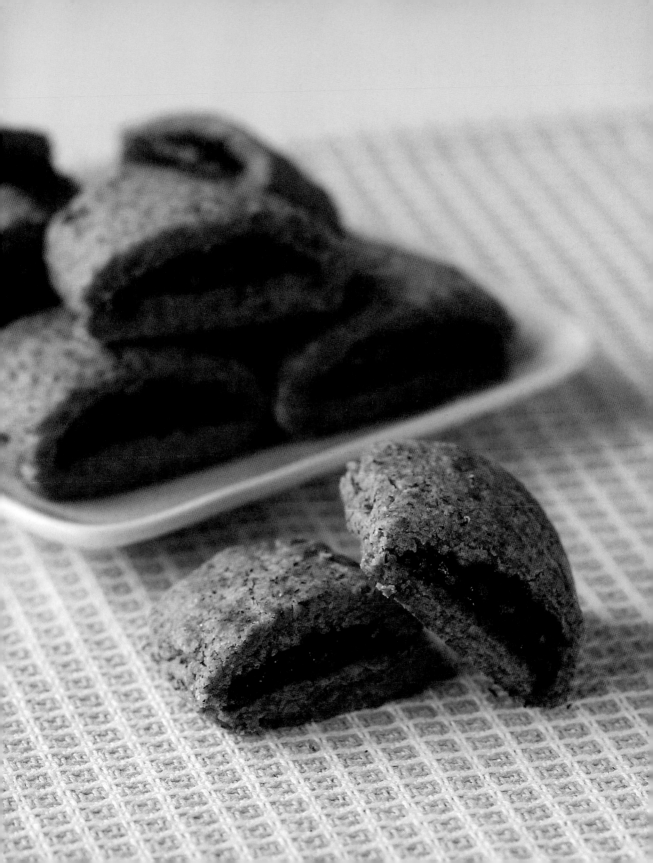

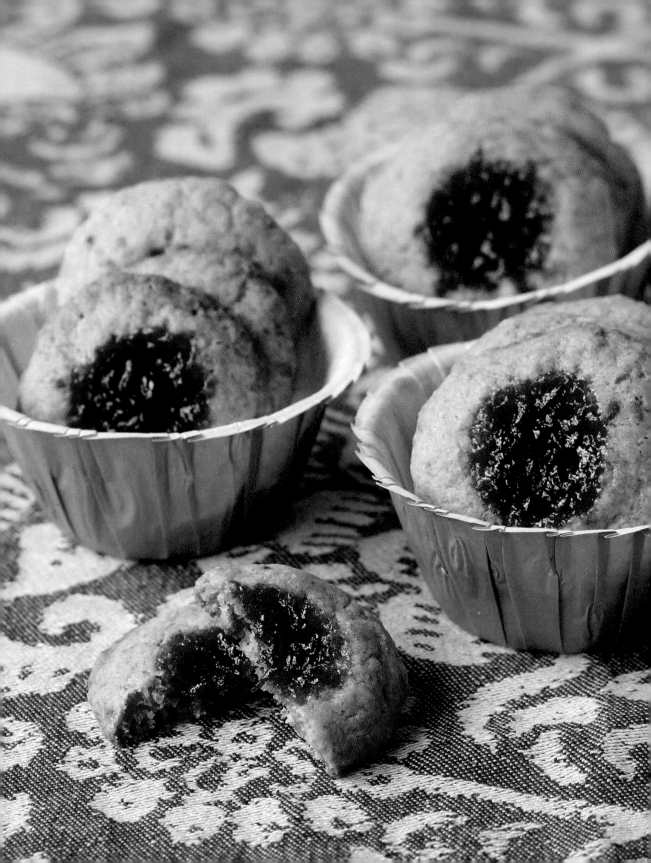

Strawberry Thumbprints

|||||||||||||||||||||||||||||||||||||||||||||||||||||||||||||||||||||||||||||||||||||||||||||||||||||||||||||||||||||||||||||||||||||||||||||||||||||||||

These cookies combine two flour blends for just the right texture. Make them with Strawberry Jam (page 82) or another favorite jam. Ask the kids to help; a child's thumb is just the right size to make thumbprints.

130 grams (about 1 cup) Pastry Flour Blend (page 24)

64 grams (about ½ cup) Basic Flour Blend (page 23)

½ teaspoon xanthan gum

1 teaspoon baking powder

½ teaspoon salt

½ cup (110 g) organic cane sugar

10 tablespoons shortening (see page 7), softened

1 Flaxseed Egg (page 42)

1 teaspoon Vanilla Extract (page 288)

¼ cup (61 g) Strawberry Jam (page 82)

1. Combine the flours, xanthan gum, baking powder, and salt in a medium bowl.
2. In a separate large bowl, cream together the sugar and shortening using a mixer on medium speed for 5 minutes, scraping down the sides of the bowl as needed. The mixture will be light and fluffy.
3. Add the flaxseed egg and vanilla. Mix for 1 minute on medium speed.
4. Slowly add in the dry ingredients and blend on medium speed, about 2 minutes. The batter will be thick. Wrap the dough tightly in plastic and chill it for an hour. Cookie dough can be refrigerated for up to 2 weeks.
5. When you are ready to make cookies preheat the oven to 350°F (180°C). Line two large baking sheets with parchment paper.
6. Use your hands to shape the dough into balls, about 1¼ inches (3 cm) round.
7. Place the cookies on the baking sheet with space in between and flatten them just slightly. Use the tip of a finger, your thumb, or the back of a small spoon to create a small well in the center of each cookie.
8. Fill the center of each cookie with ¼ teaspoon of jam.
9. Bake each sheet of cookies separately in the center of the oven for 15 to 16 minutes, until the jam centers are sizzling and the edges of the cookies are golden. Let the cookies cool on the baking sheet for 5 minutes, then transfer them to a cooling rack. Store them in an airtight container at room temperature for up to 3 days.

TO FREEZE

Baked cookies can be frozen in an airtight container for up to 3 months; thaw them at room temperature. Cookie dough (prepared through step 4) can be frozen for up to 6 months; thaw the dough in the refrigerator before forming cookies, filling with jam, and baking.

Animal Crackers

The animal crackers I remember came in a box with a ribbon handle, designed for young children to be able to carry around. My parents would buy a box for each of my siblings and me, and through a series of strategic trades my older sister usually ended up with most of the cookies in her box by the end of the day. Nostalgia aside, there's no reason why these cookies need to be saved for the kids, and there's no reason why they can't be formed into any shape you choose. Take a bite of one of these cookies and, if you're lucky, you might taste a lion or a bear.

98 grams (about ¾ cup) Pastry Flour Blend (page 24)
28 grams (about ¼ cup) gluten-free oat flour
½ teaspoon xanthan gum
¼ cup (42 g) Sucanat
½ teaspoon baking powder
¼ teaspoon salt
3 tablespoons shortening (see page 7), cold
1 tablespoon apple cider vinegar
1½ teaspoons Vanilla Extract (page 288)
Up to 2 tablespoons cold water

1. Preheat the oven to 375°F (190°C). Line a large baking sheet with parchment paper.
2. Combine the flours, xanthan gum, sugar, baking powder, and salt in a large mixing bowl.
3. Cut the shortening into tablespoon-sized pieces and lay them on top of the flour. Use a pastry cutter, a pastry fork, or your hands to work the shortening into the flour. Continue working for 3 to 4 minutes, until a crumbly mixture forms.
4. Add the vinegar, vanilla, and 1 tablespoon of water. Work the liquids into the dough. Add up to 1 tablespoon more cold water as needed, ½ tablespoon at a time, until the dough forms. (See Preparing Cookie Dough on page 236.)
5. Roll the dough between two pieces of parchment paper, about ⅜ inch (10 mm) thick. Remove the top layer of parchment and use cookie cutters to create desired shapes.
6. Remove the excess dough, roll it out again, and create additional cookies, until all of the dough is used. Arrange the cookies on the lined baking sheet. If you are using animal cookie cutters, a plastic toothpick can be used to poke holes for the eyes.
7. Bake for 9 to 10 minutes, until the tops are golden. Let the cookies cool on the baking sheet for 5 minutes, then transfer them to a cooling rack.

TO FREEZE

Baked cookies can be frozen in an airtight container for up to 3 months; thaw them at room temperature. Cookie dough (prepared through step 4) can be wrapped tightly in plastic and frozen for up to 6 months; thaw the dough in the refrigerator and bring it to room temperature before forming cookies and baking.

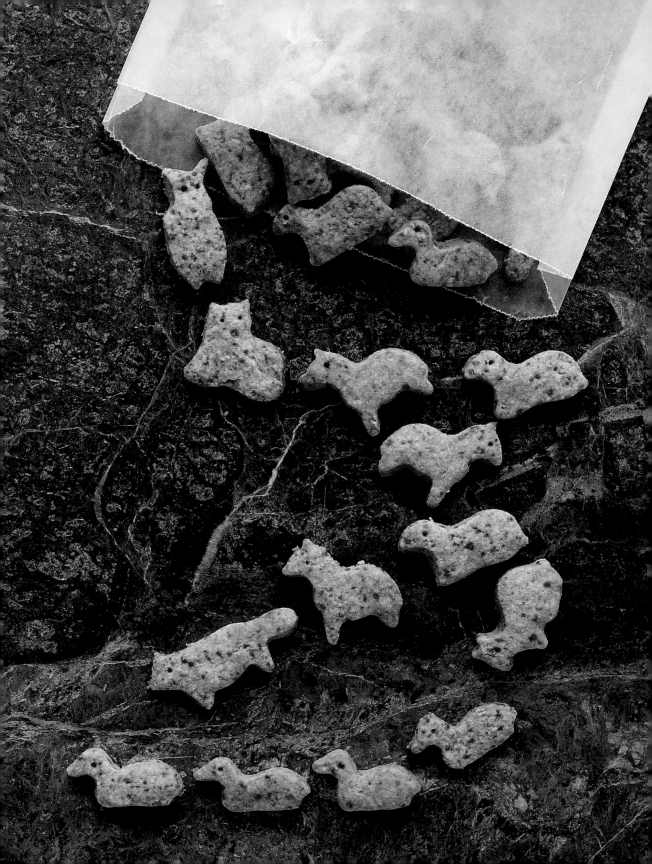

15.

Sweet
Treats

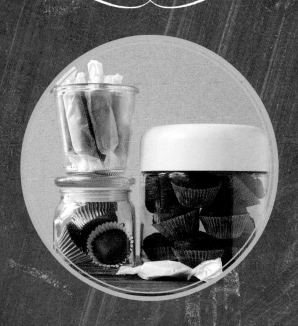

BROWNIE BITES ✑ MINI PIES ✑ BLACK-EYED BLONDIES

NON-DAIRY ICE CREAM SANDWICHES ✑ HOT COCOA ✑ CHOCOLATE

TRUFFLES ✑ SUNFLOWER BUTTER CUPS ✑ CHOCOLATE CHEWY ROLLS

RASPBERRY FRUIT ROLL-UPS ✑ CHOCOLATE PUDDING ✑ ICE POPS

Most chocolate and candies are processed in facilities that also process nuts and dairy, but there's no need to give them up completely. Bake Brownie Bites (page 255) or Black-Eyed Blondies (page 263) for a class party, or freeze Ice Pops (page 281) for a summer treat. You can end your search for a safe candy, holiday treat, or delicious cup of hot cocoa right here.

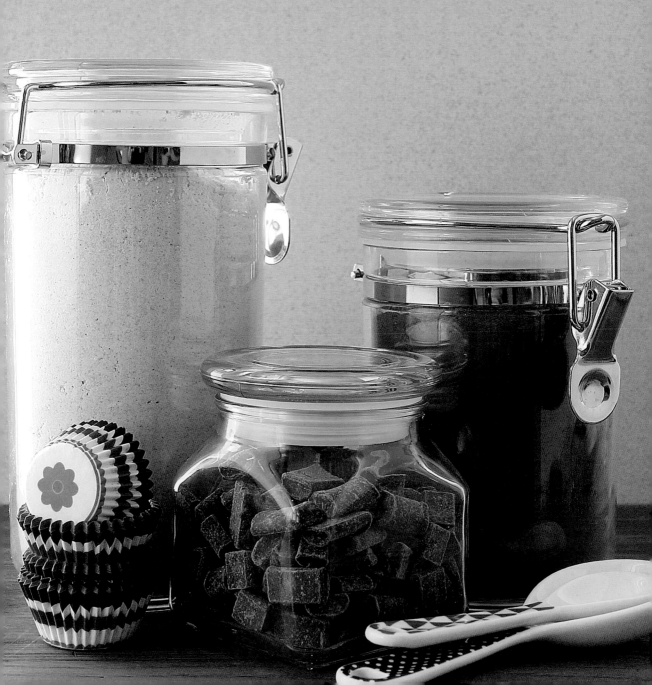

Bake

Brownie Bites

If I had my way all chocolate would be just that—luscious, dark, without too much sugar and especially without milk and nuts. My version of the traditional brownie takes on an easy bite-sized form that emphasizes the chocolate. Brownie Bites are ideal for an afternoon pick-me-up or simple dessert. If your daughter forgot to tell you about the birthday celebration at school tomorrow, top them with Vanilla Frosting (page 294) to make a stand-in for cupcakes.

64 grams (about ½ cup) Basic Flour Blend (page 23)

40 grams (about ¼ cup) buckwheat flour

¼ teaspoon xanthan gum

¼ cup (26 g) natural unsweetened cocoa powder

½ teaspoon baking powder

¼ teaspoon salt

⅓ cup plus 1 tablespoon (87 g) organic cane sugar

¼ cup plus 2 tablespoons (90 g) Applesauce (page 45)

¼ cup (60 ml) chocolate Hemp Milk (see pages 31 and 33) or non-dairy chocolate milk of choice

1 teaspoon Vanilla Extract (page 288)

¼ to ½ cup (60 to 120 g) mini chocolate chips

¼ cup (60 ml) grapeseed oil

1. Preheat the oven to 350°F (180°C). Grease the cups of a mini-muffin pan.
2. Combine the flours, xanthan gum, cocoa powder, baking powder, salt, and sugar in a bowl.
3. In a large bowl, combine the applesauce, chocolate milk, and vanilla using a mixer on medium speed for about 1 minute.
4. Melt ¼ cup (60 g) of chocolate chips together with the oil in a microwave for 20 to 30 seconds. Stir the mixture together completely, ensuring that all of the chocolate is melted.
5. Add the chocolate mixture to the wet ingredients and blend on medium speed for about 2 minutes.
6. Add the dry ingredients and blend on medium-high speed until smooth, about 2 minutes. The batter will be thick.
7. Stir in an additional ¼ cup (60 g) of chocolate chips, if desired, by hand.
8. Spoon the batter into the cups of the prepared mini-muffin pan, no more than three-quarters full.
9. Bake for 14 to 15 minutes, until a toothpick inserted comes out clean. Allow the brownie bites to cool for 10 to 15 minutes in the pan before transferring them to a cooling rack. Store them in an airtight container at room temperature for 3 to 4 days.

TO FREEZE

Freeze Brownie Bites in an airtight container for up to 6 months. Thaw them at room temperature before serving.

A NOTE ABOUT PAPER LINERS

I don't recommend paper liners when baking with gluten-free grains, as they have a tendency to hold in moisture. Instead, bake directly in the muffin pan and add the paper cups, if desired, after cooling.

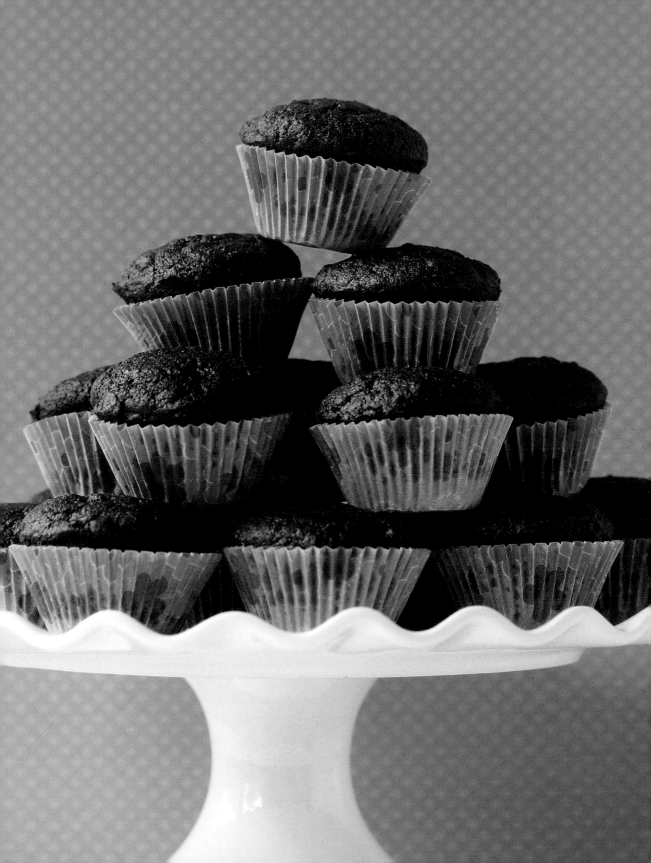

Mini Pies

Whether you are baking for a crowd and want to impress your guests with their own miniature pies—or simply need individual portions—this recipe will do the trick. The cups of a standard-sized muffin pan act as the pie plate.

Fill the pies with either of the two options I offer for you here—blueberry or apple—or choose your favorite pie filling. The ingredients listed here are for 8 pies. If you choose to make a mixed batch of 4 blueberry pies and 4 apple pies, halve both sets of filling ingredients.

FOR THE CRUST

260 grams (about 2 cups) Pastry Flour Blend (page 24)

½ teaspoon xanthan gum

¼ cup (55 g) organic cane sugar

½ teaspoon salt

8 tablespoons shortening (see page 7), cold

2 tablespoons apple cider vinegar

¼ cup (60 ml) plus 1 tablespoon cold water

Up to 3 tablespoons additional flour for dusting

FOR BLUEBERRY FILLING (8 MINI PIES)

1½ cups (225 g) blueberries

2 teaspoons lemon zest

2 teaspoons fresh lemon juice

2 tablespoons tapioca starch

3 tablespoons organic cane sugar

½ teaspoon ground cinnamon

FOR APPLE FILLING (8 MINI PIES)

1½ cups (150 g) peeled, cored, and diced apples (about 2 apples)

¼ cup (40 g) raisins, optional

1 tablespoon fresh lemon juice

2 tablespoons tapioca starch

¼ cup (55 g) organic cane sugar

½ teaspoon ground cinnamon

FOR TOPPING

2 tablespoons turbinado sugar, optional

To prepare the crust

1. Combine the flour, xanthan gum, ¼ cup (55 g) cane sugar, and salt in a large mixing bowl.

2. Cut the shortening into tablespoon-sized pieces and lay them on top of the flour. Use a pastry cutter, a pastry fork, or your hands to work the shortening into the flour. Continue working for 3 to 4 minutes, until a crumbly mixture forms.

3. Add the vinegar and ¼ cup (60 ml) water. Work the liquids into the dough using the pastry cutter. Add up to 1 more tablespoon of cold water as needed, ½ tablespoon at a time, until the dough is smooth and pliable.

4. Separate the dough into three sections (to make it easier to work with later) and form each section into a disk, about ½ inch (13 mm) thick. Wrap the disks tightly in plastic and refrigerate for 30 minutes. Pastry dough can be refrigerated for up to 2 weeks.

5. When you are ready to make the pies, preheat the oven to 350°F (180°C). Grease 8 cups of a 12-cup standard muffin pan.

(recipe continues)

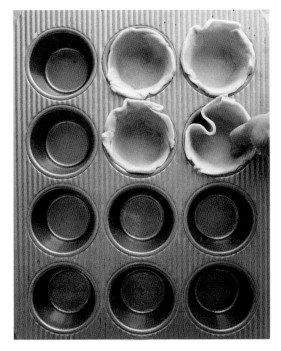

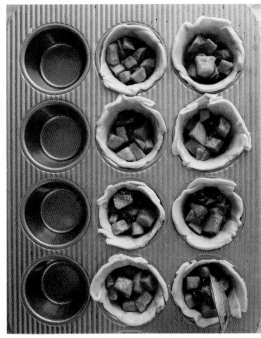

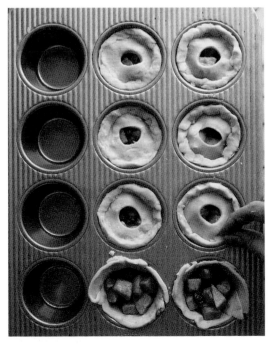

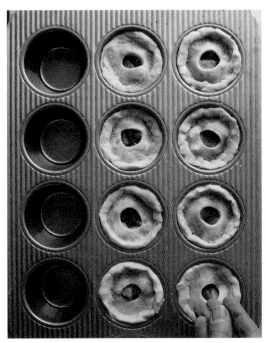

6. If the dough has been refrigerated for more than 30 minutes prior to rolling, let it sit at room temperature for 15 minutes and massage it with your hands until it is pliable. Roll out the dough between two sheets of parchment paper. Use additional flour, if needed, to avoid sticking.

7. Cut eight 4½-inch (11.5 cm) rounds to form the bottom crusts. Use two of the three sections of dough for this step. Place the bottom crusts into the wells of the prepared muffin pan. The pastry should fully cover the bottom and sides of the wells with up to ¼ inch (6.5 mm) of crust protruding from the wells.

8. Roll out the remaining section of dough and cut eight 2½-inch (6.5 cm) rounds for the top crusts. Cut a ⅞-inch (2 cm) center hole in the top crusts.

To make the filling (either blueberry or apple)

9. Toss the fruit (blueberries and zest or apples and raisins) with lemon juice in a small bowl.

10. Combine the starch, remaining cane sugar, and cinnamon in a separate bowl. Add this to the fruit, and toss to coat.

11. Distribute the fruit evenly in the bottom crusts.

To finish the pies

12. Place the top crusts over the fruit, allowing them to sit inside the bottom crusts. Use your fingers to roll and pinch the edges together.

13. Sprinkle turbinado sugar on the tops of the crusts, if desired.

14. Bake for 19 to 20 minutes, until the fruit filling is bubbling and the tops are golden.

TO FREEZE

Freeze pie dough (prepared through step 4) for up to 6 months; thaw the dough in the refrigerator and then let it sit at room temperature for 15 minutes before rolling, filling, and baking. Pies are best when freshly baked, but they can be frozen in an airtight container for up to 2 months; thaw them in the refrigerator and reheat at 325°F (165°C) for 12 to 13 minutes, until warm.

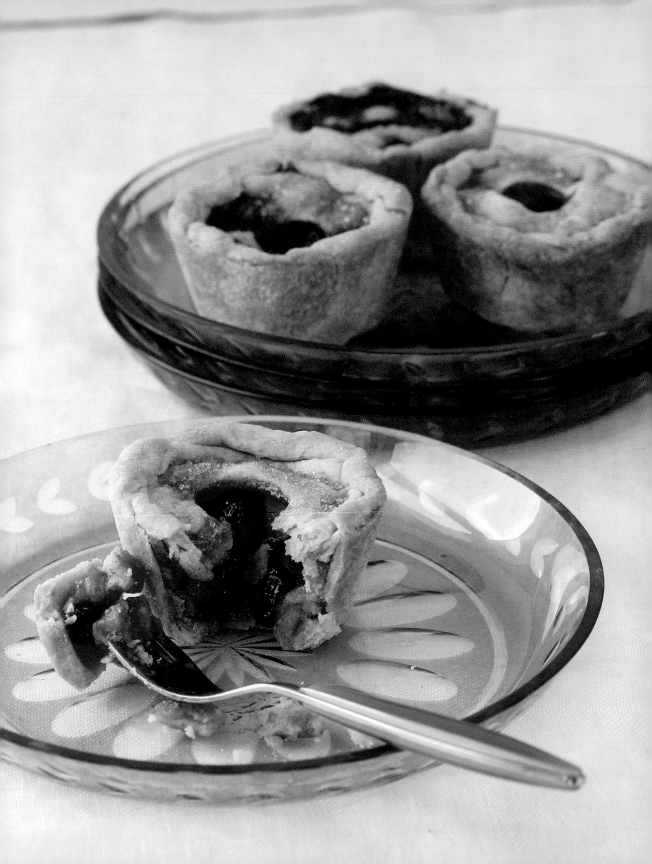

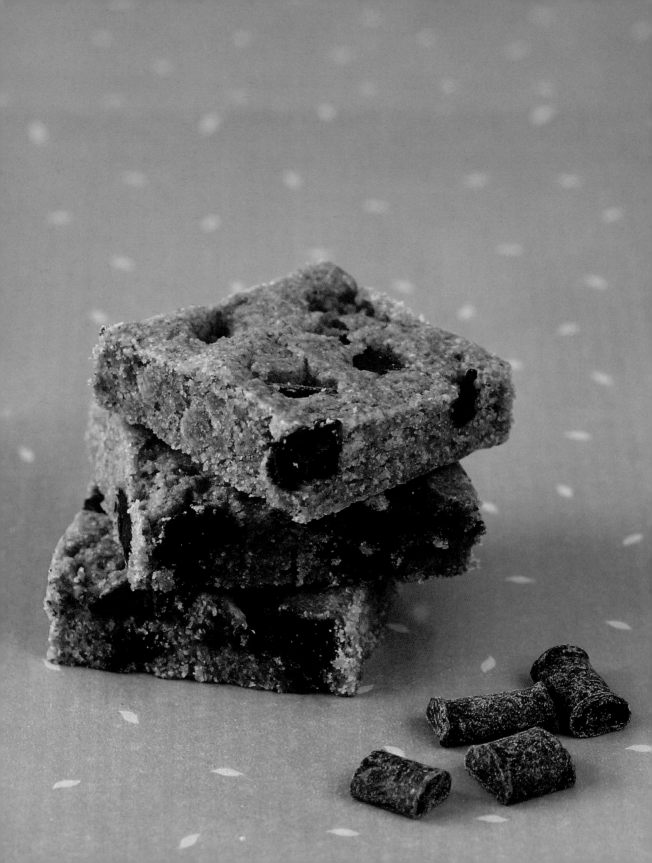

Black-Eyed Blondies

*B*londies were one of my grandmother's favorite treats to make. They made regular appearances in care packages at college, and she always had a batch in her freezer for company. I had to reinvent my grandmother's recipe dozens of times before I achieved a blondie that tastes just like a favorite chocolate chip cookie, with the texture of a fudgy brownie. They are half cookie and half brownie but all good.

Put the electric mixer away; this recipe is made by hand.

192 grams (about 1½ cups) Basic Flour Blend (page 23)

½ teaspoon xanthan gum

½ teaspoon baking powder

¼ teaspoon salt

¾ cup (108 g) organic light brown sugar

8 tablespoons shortening, melted

¼ cup plus 2 tablespoons (90 g) Applesauce (page 45)

1½ teaspoons Vanilla Extract (page 288)

⅓ cup (80 g) chocolate chunks or dark chocolate chips

1. Preheat the oven to 350°F (180°C). Grease a 9-inch (23 cm) square baking dish.
2. Combine the flour, xanthan gum, baking powder, and salt in a medium bowl.
3. Combine the sugar and melted shortening (while still warm) in a separate mixing bowl. Stir until the sugar is melted.
4. Add the applesauce and vanilla to the wet ingredients and stir for 20 seconds to combine.
5. Add the dry ingredients and stir by hand until the ingredients are fully blended and the batter is thick and slightly glossy.
6. Stir in the chocolate chunks, by hand.
7. Scoop the batter into the prepared baking dish and use the back of a spoon to pat it to the edges of the baking dish. Redistribute the chocolate chunks, if needed, so they aren't clumped together.
8. Bake for 22 to 24 minutes, until the top is lightly browned.
9. Cool the blondies completely before cutting them into squares. Store them in an airtight container at room temperature for 3 to 4 days.

TO FREEZE

Freeze Black-Eyed Blondies in an airtight container for up to 6 months. Thaw them at room temperature before serving.

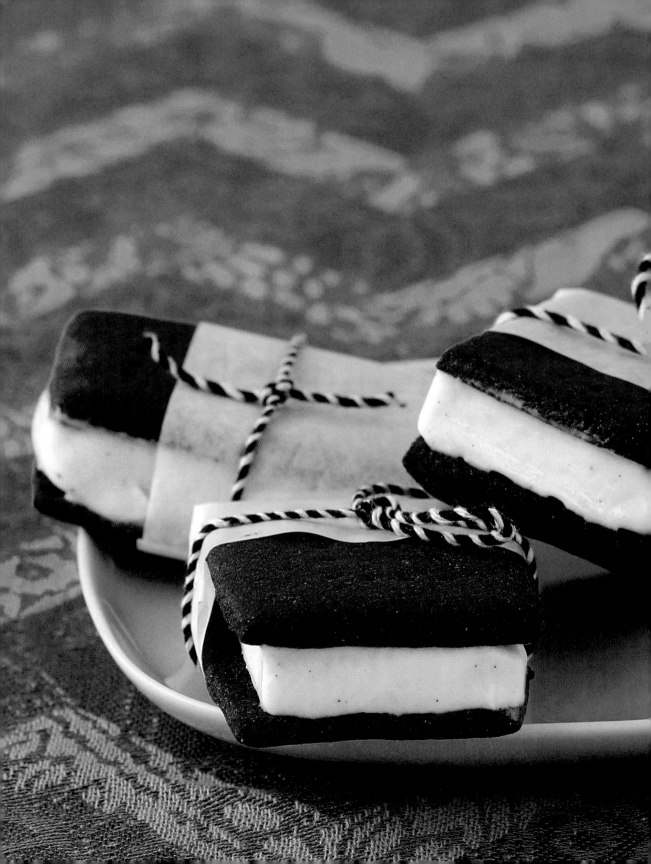

Non-Dairy
Ice Cream Sandwiches

MAKES 8 SANDWICHES

*N*othing says summer more than a chocolate sandwich cookie filled with vanilla ice cream. Use your favorite non-dairy frozen dessert to make this allergen-free treat; two of my favorite brands are Living Harvest Foods Tempt (made from hemp milk) and So Delicious Coconut Milk Frozen Desserts. Be sure to check the labels and choose one that is safe for you and your family.

160 grams (about 1¼ cups) Basic Flour Blend (page 23)

½ teaspoon xanthan gum

½ cup (52 g) natural unsweetened cocoa powder

½ cup (110 g) organic cane sugar

2 teaspoons baking powder

¼ teaspoon salt

8 tablespoons shortening (see page 7), melted

3 tablespoons chocolate Hemp Milk (page 31) or non-dairy chocolate milk of choice

1 tablespoon Applesauce (page 45)

1 teaspoon Vanilla Extract (page 288)

1 pint (473 ml) of your favorite allergen-free frozen dessert

1. Preheat the oven to 350°F (180°C). Line two large baking sheets with parchment paper.

2. Combine the flour, xanthan gum, cocoa powder, sugar, baking powder, and salt in a medium bowl.

3. In a large bowl, blend together the shortening, milk, applesauce, and vanilla using a mixer on medium speed for 1 minute.

4. Add the dry ingredients and mix on medium speed until combined. Mix for another 2 minutes on medium-high speed until the dough forms a glossy ball.

5. Roll out the dough between two sheets of parchment to about a ⅛-inch (3 mm) thickness. Use a sharp knife to cut 16 rectangular cookies, 2 inches (5 cm) wide by 3 inches (7.5 cm) long.

6. Place the cookies on the prepared baking sheets with space in between. Use a fork to pierce holes in the cookies.

7. Bake each sheet separately for 12 to 13 minutes in the center of the oven. Let the cookies cool completely and then freeze them in an airtight container for at least two hours.

8. Sandwiches can be assembled a few at a time or all at once. Let the frozen dessert stand at room temperature for about 10 minutes, until it is just soft around the edges.

9. Release the frozen dessert from the container onto a large cutting board. Use a sharp knife to cut it into rectangles the same size as the cookies, about ⅜ inch (10 mm) thick.

(recipe continues)

10. Assemble the sandwiches with a cookie on bottom, a layer of frozen dessert in the center, and a cookie on top. Press gently to secure them.

11. Place the sandwiches back into the freezer-safe container and freeze for at least an hour before serving.

TO FREEZE

Once assembled, the sandwiches will be best eaten within 1 week. The cookies can be frozen in an airtight container (without the ice cream filling) for up to 6 months.

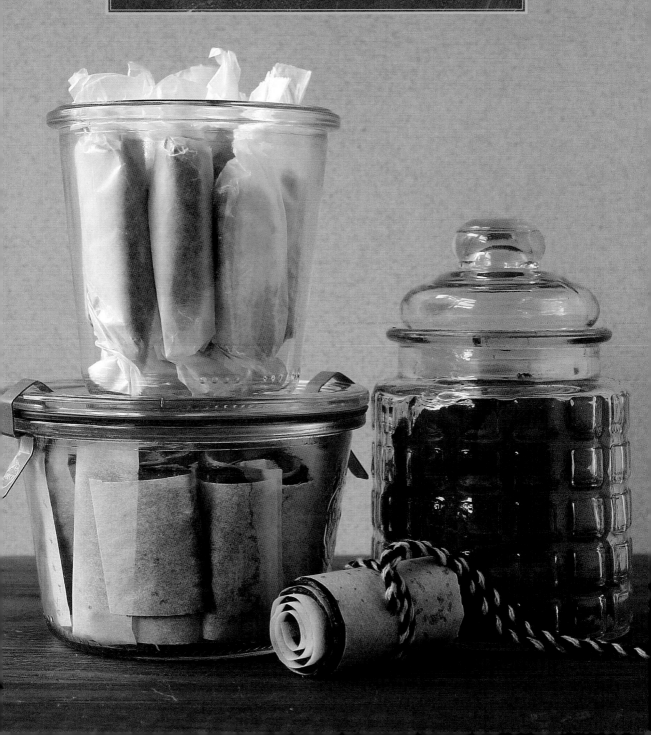

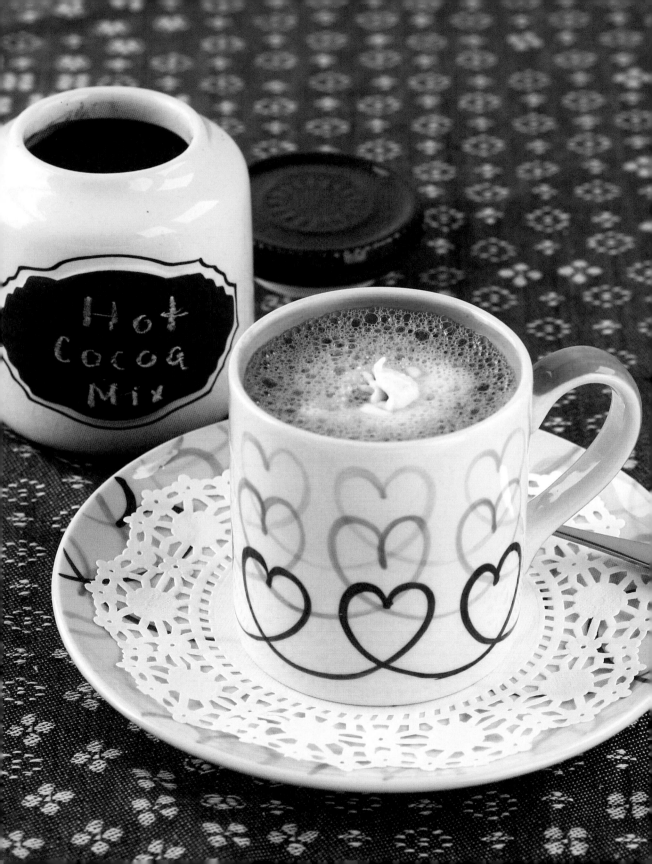

Hot Cocoa

Hot Cocoa is meant for snow days, and yes—it's quite easy to make, even without dairy. Choose your favorite non-dairy milk, heat it up, and stir in some of this cocoa mix. Store the mix in the pantry for up to 2 months—just long enough to get you through the coldest winter months. The cinnamon is optional, but I urge you to try it (unless you are allergic to cinnamon) as it really makes the Hot Cocoa special. Add a dollop of Whipped Coconut Cream (page 35), if desired.

FOR THE COCOA MIX

1 cup (220 g) organic cane sugar

¾ cup (78 g) natural unsweetened cocoa powder

⅛ teaspoon salt

⅛ teaspoon ground cinnamon, optional

FOR THE HOT COCOA (ONE SERVING)

1 to 1½ cups (240 to 360 ml) Hemp Milk (page 31) or non-dairy milk of choice

2 to 3 tablespoons Cocoa Mix

To make the mix

1. Whisk together the sugar, cocoa powder, salt, and cinnamon, if desired. Store the cocoa mix in the pantry in an airtight container.

To make hot cocoa

2. Heat the milk in a small saucepan over medium-low heat. Use 1 cup (240 ml) of milk per 8-ounce serving, or 1½ cups (360 ml) of milk per 12-ounce serving.

3. Stir in 2 tablespoons of hot cocoa mix per 8-ounce serving or 3 tablespoons of hot cocoa mix per 12-ounce serving.

Chocolate Truffles

MAKES ABOUT 24 TRUFFLES

*S*urprise your kids or your honey on Valentine's Day with these truffles instead of the chocolates in the red heart boxes. This recipe transforms chocolate chips into decadent truffles, ideal for any special day or for a hostess gift.

1½ tablespoons shortening (see page 7)
¼ cup (60 ml) coconut milk creamer
1 cup (240 g) chocolate chips
½ teaspoon Vanilla Extract (page 288)
¼ cup (26 g) natural unsweetened cocoa powder

1. Melt the shortening over low heat in a small saucepan. Add the coconut milk creamer. Increase the heat to medium and bring just to a boil, stirring occasionally.

2. Remove the saucepan from the heat and stir in the chocolate chips and vanilla. Stir vigorously until the mixture is smooth and glossy.

3. Transfer the chocolate to a large mixing bowl and refrigerate it for up to an hour and a half, until it is hardened but still pliable. Soften it using the paddle attachment of a mixer, for about 20 seconds on low speed.

4. Scoop out small portions of chocolate, about 2 teaspoons (or desired size), and place them on a sheet of parchment paper. Use cool, dry hands to roll each chocolate into a ball using very light pressure. If your hands start to get too warm or the chocolate starts to soften, refrigerate the chocolates for a few minutes and start again.

5. Place the cocoa powder in a shallow dish. Roll the truffles in the cocoa powder, to lightly coat them on all sides. Refrigerate the truffles in an airtight container for up to 2 weeks.

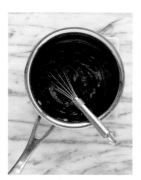 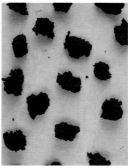 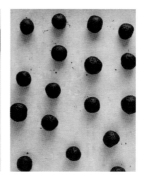 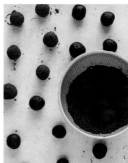

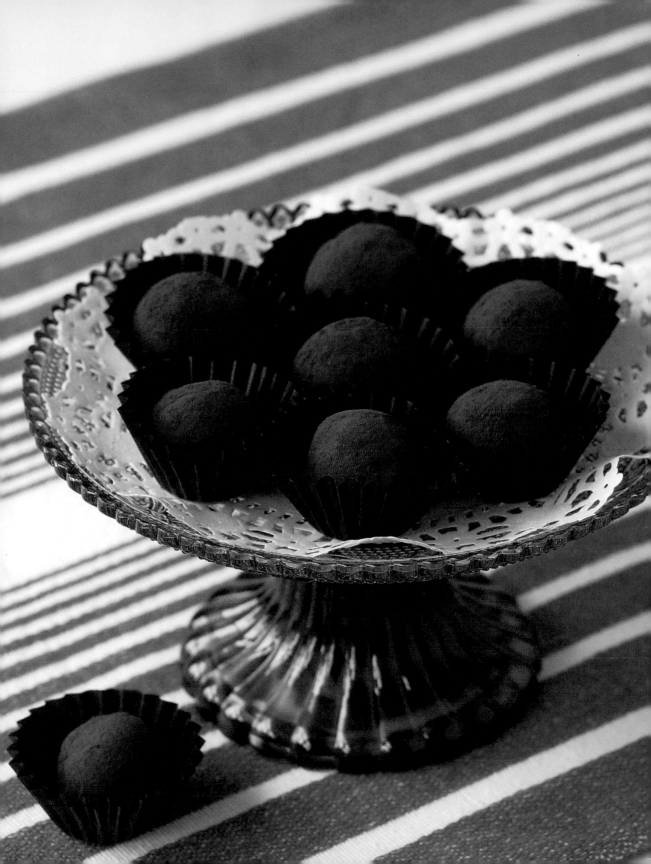

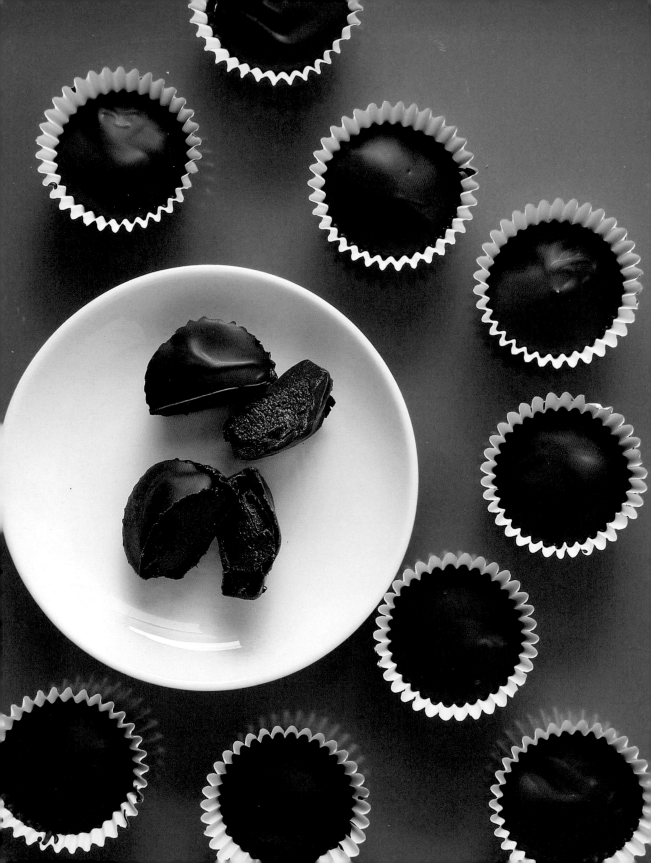

Sunflower Butter Cups

MAKES 24 MINI CUPS

These luscious treats mimic traditional peanut butter cups and are a lot of fun to make. Sweeten them up by adding more sugar while preparing the Sunflower Seed Butter (page 77) or fill them with Chocolate Sunflower Butter (page 78) to satisfy hard-core chocoholics.

1 tablespoon shortening (see page 7)
2 cups (480 g) chocolate chips
¾ cup (175 g) Sunflower Seed Butter (page 77)

1. Fill the cups of a 24-cup mini-muffin pan with foil liners. The pan provides additional structure.

2. Melt the shortening over low heat. Add the chocolate chips and stir continuously until the chocolate is completely melted.

3. Drop a small amount of melted chocolate (about 2 teaspoons) in the bottom of each liner. Work the chocolate halfway up the edges of the liners by carefully rolling the chocolate in each liner. Place the coated liners back in the muffin pan and refrigerate for 15 minutes.

4. Add the sunflower seed butter in the center of the cups, using about ½ tablespoon per cup.

5. Spoon the remaining chocolate on top of the butter, allowing it to seep down the sides to meet the bottom chocolate layer.

6. Refrigerate the candies for at least an hour before serving, and up to 2 months. They are best kept refrigerated until an hour or two before serving; they will melt in warm weather and in your hands.

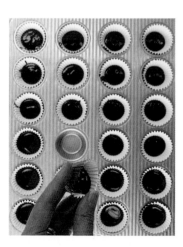 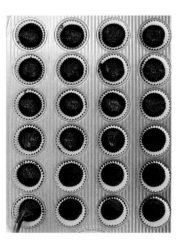 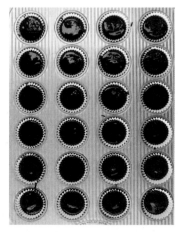

Chocolate Chewy Rolls

MAKES ABOUT 24 CANDIES

Sometimes a safe lollipop just doesn't do the trick. That's where these chocolate candies that replace the traditional Tootsie Roll come in. They are a wonderful trade for Halloween candies, or to hide in an Easter egg. As a bonus, this no-bake treat is fun to make with the kids.

¼ cup plus 2 tablespoons (39 g) natural unsweetened cocoa powder

¼ cup (36 g) Powdered Sugar (page 286)

1¼ cups (190 g) powdered rice milk

½ cup (120 ml) honey

1 tablespoon shortening (see page 7), melted

1 teaspoon Vanilla Extract (page 288)

1. Combine the cocoa, powdered sugar, and ½ cup (76 g) of powdered rice milk in a medium bowl. Mix the ingredients together well and set it aside. This will be a very powdery mixture.

2. In a large bowl, blend together the honey, shortening, and vanilla using a mixer on medium speed for about 1 minute.

3. Add the dry ingredients, one third at a time, and blend on low speed until completely combined, about 5 minutes. Add up to ¼ cup (38 g) more powdered rice milk, if needed, until a thick candy dough ball forms.

4. Spread 2 tablespoons of rice milk on a smooth prep surface. Place the candy dough ball on top.

5. Work the remaining powdered milk into the candy ball with your hands, a little bit at a time by flattening the ball, adding powdered rice milk, massaging it into the dough with your hands, and rolling it into a ball. Repeat this process until you have used all of the rice milk or you can no longer manipulate the ball with your hands.

6. Flatten the candy ball into a ½-inch (13 mm) thick rectangle. Let it rest for 20 to 30 minutes.

7. Use a sharp nonstick knife to cut the candies into desired size pieces. Roll them in any remaining powdered rice milk.

8. Cut twenty-four 3-inch (7.5 cm) squares of wax paper. Wrap the candies individually in the papers and store them at room temperature for up to 2 months.

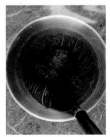 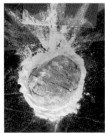 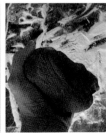 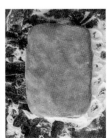 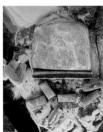

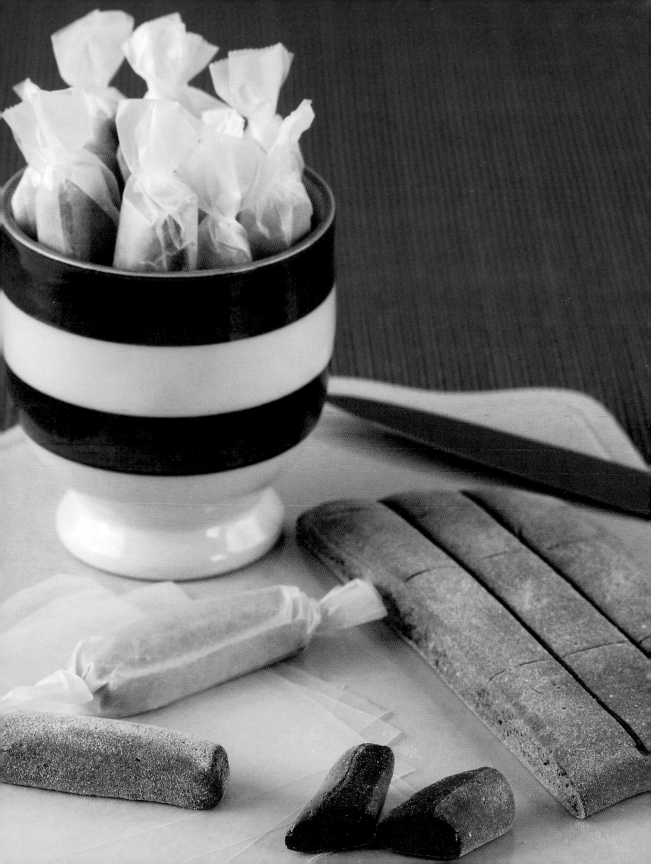

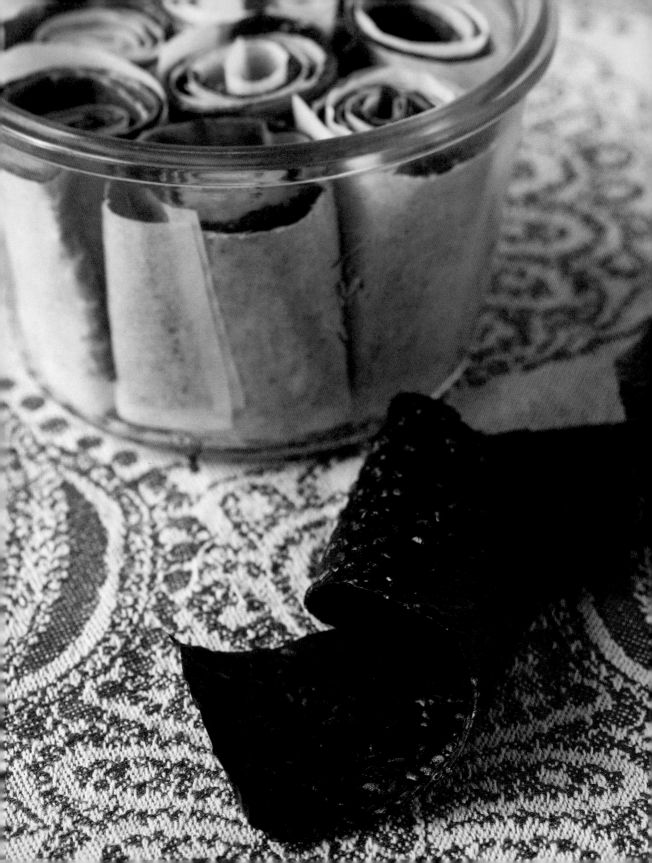

Raspberry Fruit Roll-Ups

MAKES 8 ROLLS

Fruit roll-ups are a great healthy snack, but off-the-shelf versions often contain preservatives and food colorings that you may prefer to avoid. This recipe takes up to 2 days (elapsed time) to make, but requires very little attention. If you have a food dehydrator, this is the time to use it; otherwise, use your oven. Add up to ¼ cup (55 g) more sugar for a sweeter version.

3 cups (372 g) raspberries
3 tablespoons organic cane sugar
1 tablespoon fresh lemon juice
1 tablespoon lemon zest

1. Puree the fruit in a food processor or blender.
2. Combine the pureed fruit, sugar, lemon juice, and zest in a medium non-reactive saucepan. Bring to a boil over medium heat. Turn the heat to medium-low and cook for 12 to 15 minutes, stirring occasionally, until the mixture is reduced by half.
3. If you are using a dehydrator, follow the instructions for your machine. Otherwise preheat the oven to 200°F (95°C). Line a large baking sheet with parchment paper.
4. Spread the fruit mixture on the baking sheet in a uniformly thick layer, working to within 1 inch (2.5 cm) of the edges. Turn the oven off and place the baking sheet in the oven to dehydrate.
5. Every 6 to 8 hours check the roll-ups for doneness. Reheat the oven to 200°F (95°C) and turn it off. Repeat this step as many times as needed, until the fruit is tacky. If you need to use the oven during this process, remove the baking sheet, then replace it once the oven has cooled down to about 200°F (95°C).
6. When the fruit is tacky and you are able to peel the edges, the roll-ups are ready to cut. Place a second piece of parchment on top of the fruit. Cut 8 ribbons of fruit and roll them. Refrigerate leftover roll-ups in an airtight container for up to 2 weeks.

Chocolate Pudding

Chocolate pudding is the ultimate comfort food—smooth, creamy, and chocolaty, of course. Sore throats, bruised knees, and bruised egos will all feel better after a spoonful of this pudding.

3 tablespoons corn starch

2 cups (480 ml) coconut milk beverage or non-dairy milk of choice, at room temperature

⅓ cup (73 g) organic cane sugar

¼ cup (26 g) natural unsweetened cocoa powder

⅛ teaspoon salt

1 teaspoon Vanilla Extract (page 288)

¼ cup (60 g) chocolate chips

1. Whisk the corn starch and ½ cup (120 ml) of milk together in a small bowl, making sure there are no lumps.

2. Combine the sugar, cocoa powder, and salt in a separate medium bowl.

3. Warm the remaining milk and vanilla in a medium saucepan over low heat for 2 to 3 minutes. Whisk in the cocoa mixture, stirring until the milk is smooth. Add the chocolate chips and continue heating over low heat, whisking until the chocolate chips are completely melted.

4. Increase the heat to medium-high, and bring to a boil, without stirring.

5. As soon as the mixture starts to boil, decrease the heat to low, and briskly whisk in the corn starch mixture (from step 1). The pudding will thicken. Continue to heat for 1 minute longer, stirring constantly.

6. Let the pudding cool for 15 minutes, then spoon it into four serving cups. Cover the serving cups with plastic wrap, allowing the plastic to sit directly on the pudding (so that it won't create a skin). Refrigerate for at least 2 hours before serving or up to a week.

TO SUBSTITUTE

For a corn-free version substitute tapioca starch for corn starch.

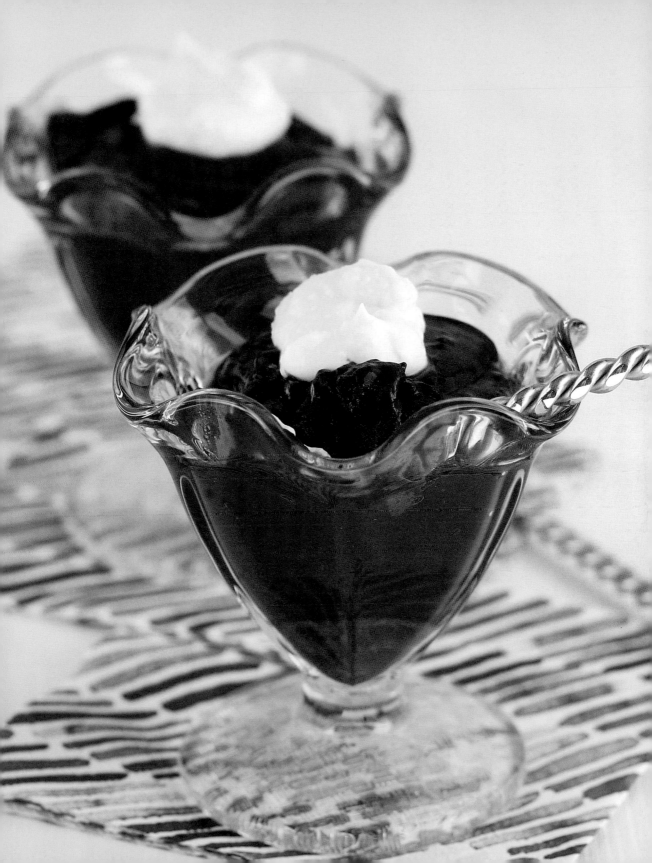

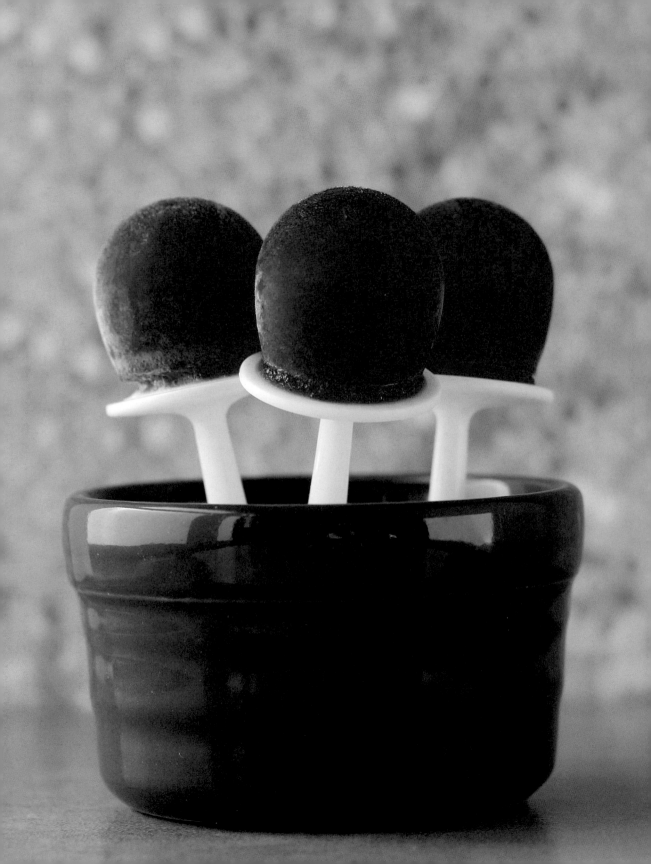

Ice Pops

These frozen treats are almost as easy to make as ice cubes. This recipe combines the flavors of strawberry and lemon to cool you off on a hot summer day, but feel free to switch up the fruit and juice. If you have leftover juice after filling the ice pop molds, freeze it in ice cube trays; the resulting strawberry lemonade ice cubes turn iced tea or seltzer into a refreshing summer drink.

Vary the fruit and the juice to create new flavors and avoid your food allergens; pair different berries or pureed fruits with any juice. Adjust the sugar to your taste and the tartness of the ingredients you choose.

¼ cup (55 g) organic cane sugar

1 cup (240 ml) water

¾ cup (105 g) strawberries, hulled and chopped

½ cup (120 ml) fresh lemon juice

1. Combine the sugar and ½ cup (120 ml) of water in a small saucepan and bring to a boil over medium-high heat. Remove the pan from the heat, stir in the remaining water, and refrigerate for 15 minutes.

2. Puree the strawberries and lemon juice together in a food processor or blender. Add the chilled sugar water and blend for 30 seconds.

3. Pour the mixture into ice pop molds. Place the sticks into the molds and freeze for approximately 6 to 8 hours, following the directions for your ice pop molds. These will keep in the freezer for up to 3 months.

16.

Sugar *and* More

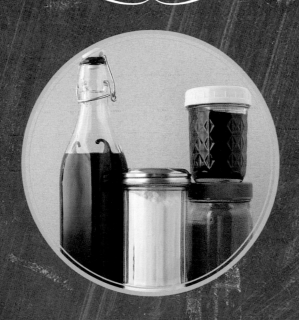

POWDERED SUGAR ⚯ CINNAMON SUGAR ⚯ VANILLA EXTRACT

CARAMEL SAUCE ⚯ CHOCOLATE SYRUP ⚯ VANILLA FROSTING

NATURAL FOOD COLORINGS

Ah, the sweet stuff. While it is usually possible to find safe off-the-shelf sugar options—and you are welcome to use them if you prefer—you may be concerned about the ingredients in food coloring or need a corn-free powdered sugar. Whether it's creamy Vanilla Frosting (page 294) with Natural Food Colorings (page 296) for a special cake or Caramel Sauce (page 291) to top your frozen dessert sundae, the simple recipes in this chapter will help you finish it off.

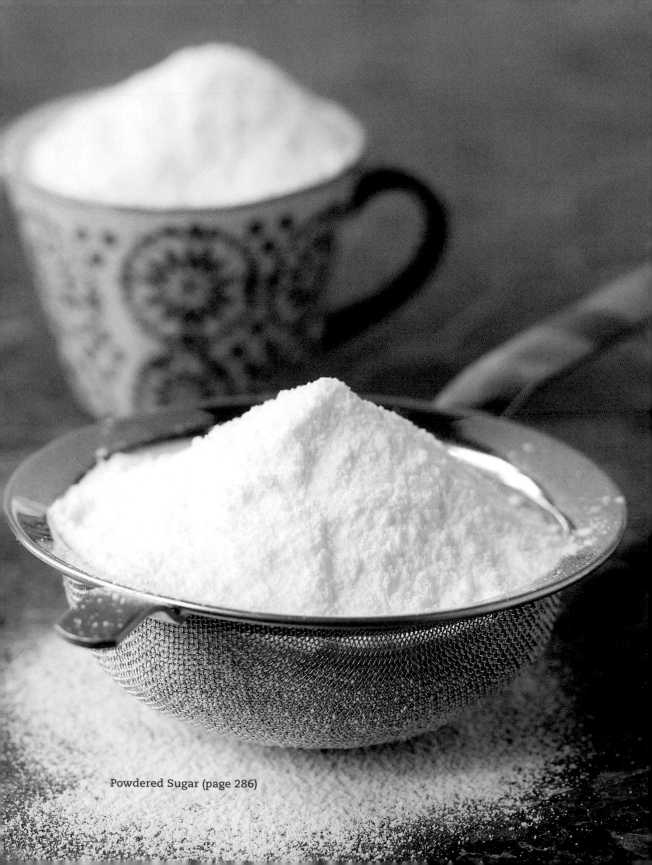

Powdered Sugar (page 286)

Powdered Sugar

MAKES 1½ CUPS (220 G)

Powdered sugar or confectioners' sugar is nothing more than finely milled sugar with a bit of starch added to prevent clumping. Most often the starch used in commercially available confectioners' sugar is corn starch—a concern for those with corn allergies. This version can be made completely starch-free (if you plan to use it today) or with your choice of starch (see page 21). It is best made in small batches to achieve an even texture. If you have a dry container for your blender, use it here.

When a recipe calls for Powdered Sugar you may substitute any off-the-shelf confectioners' sugar that is safe for you.

1 cup (220 g) granulated cane sugar

¾ teaspoon arrowroot or tapioca starch, optional

TO SUBSTITUTE

Organic cane sugar can be substituted for granulated cane sugar; the color will be off-white.

1. Combine the sugar and starch, if desired, in a food processor or blender and mix on medium-high speed for 30 seconds.
2. Scrape down the sides of the bowl and mix again until a powdery texture is reached. Store it in an airtight container in the pantry.

Cinnamon Sugar

MAKES ½ CUP (112 G)

For the days (and the recipes) when just plain sugar isn't enough, mix up a batch of Cinnamon Sugar. Don't save this just for Snickerdoodles (page 245); try some in your morning coffee too!

½ cup (110 g) organic cane sugar

1 tablespoon ground cinnamon

Mix the sugar and cinnamon together well, breaking up any clumps of cinnamon. Store it in an airtight container in the pantry.

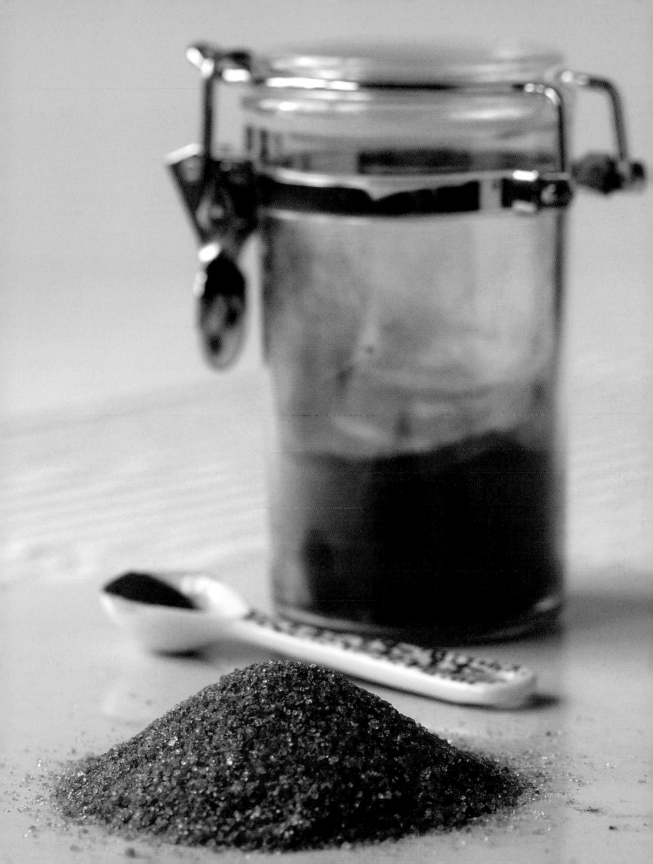

Vanilla Extract

There's no need to search for gluten-free vanilla extract at the grocery store when you can make it at home. The most common alcohols used to make vanilla extract are vodka and bourbon. While some experts argue that there is none of the grain left in distilled alcohol, your doctor may advise you not to choose alcohol derived from a grain you are allergic to.

Many vodkas are made from potatoes, but some are made from wheat or rye. Bourbon must be at least 51 percent derived from corn, which means the other 49 percent can be made from other grains—usually wheat, barley, and/or rye, the gluten grains. Those with gluten or wheat allergies should choose vodka made from potatoes or 100 percent corn bourbon. Government rules for labeling alcohol differ from those for food; check with the manufacturer to make sure the alcohol you choose is safe for you.

1½ cups (360 ml) gluten-free bourbon or vodka

3 whole vanilla beans

1. Pour the alcohol into a tall, medium-sized bottle or jar with a lid.
2. Use a sharp knife to score the vanilla beans from top to bottom, without slicing all the way through; this will allow the seeds to be released from the pods. Place the vanilla beans (with the seeds) in the jar with the alcohol. Seal the jar and shake.
3. Let the vanilla extract sit in the pantry, shaking every few days, for at least five weeks before using it.
4. When the vanilla extract is complete, fish out the vanilla beans. Save them for use in jams and other recipes that call for vanilla beans (e.g., Strawberry Jam, page 82, or Cherry Vanilla Jam, page 89).

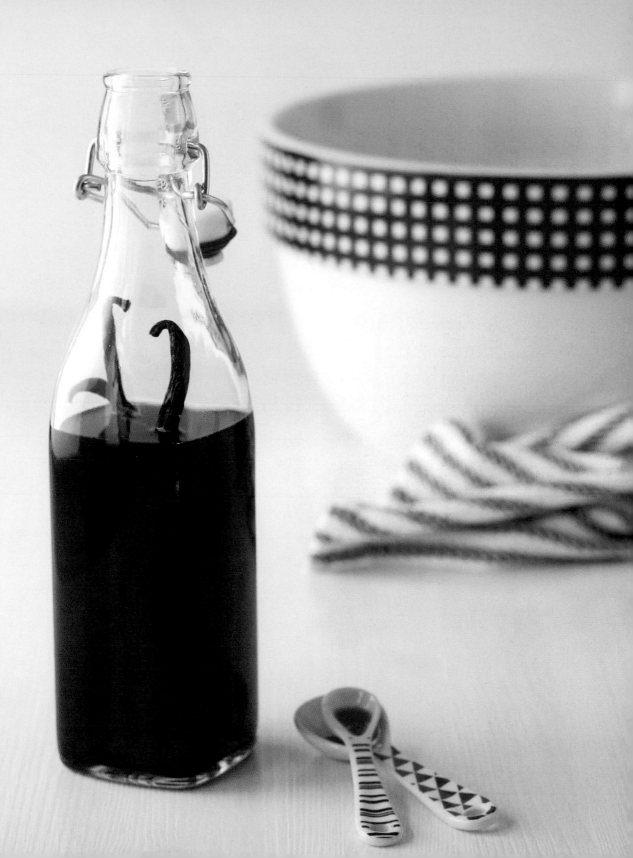

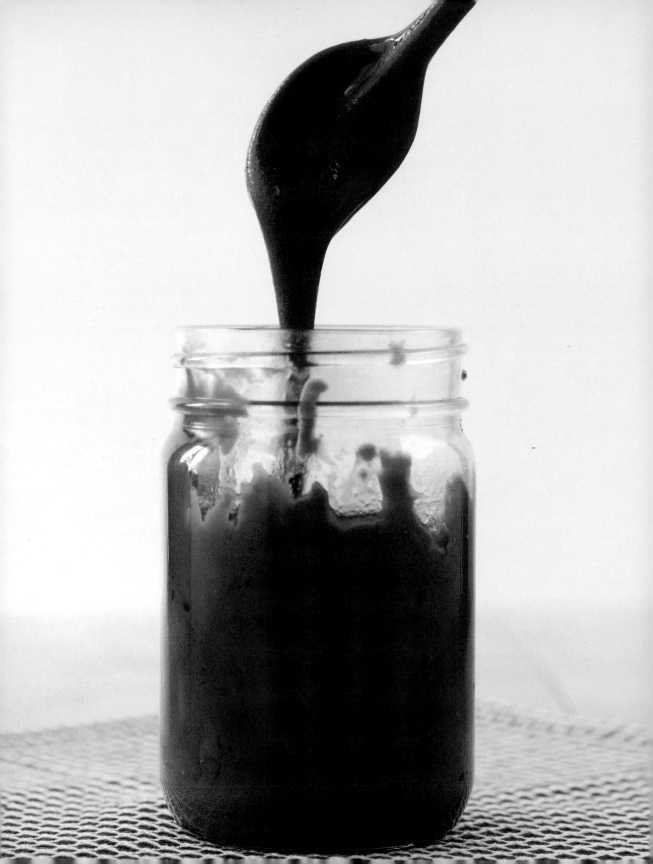

Caramel Sauce

Caramel sauce is a mixture of sugar, cooked until it's caramelized, and cream. I use coconut milk creamer in my version, instead of the heavy cream traditional recipes call for. Ooey, gooey, that's caramel.

5 tablespoons shortening (see page 7)
½ cup (120 ml) coconut milk creamer (see page 33)
1½ teaspoons Vanilla Extract (page 288)
1 cup (220 g) organic cane sugar
¼ cup (60 ml) brown rice syrup
2 tablespoons water

1. Melt 4 tablespoons of the shortening in a small saucepan over low heat. Remove the pan from the heat and add the creamer and vanilla. Stir well.

2. Combine the sugar, syrup, and water in a separate medium saucepan with high sides. Stir the ingredients together over low heat, until the sugar is melted. Increase the heat to medium-low and bring it to a low boil. Let it boil, without stirring, for about 20 minutes, until the mixture is medium golden brown.

3. Remove the sugar from the heat and stir in the cream mixture. As you do this, the sauce will bubble intensely. Stand back, and use an oven mitt to protect your hand. Stir the sauce until it is smooth.

4. Return the pot to medium-low heat and simmer for another 8 to 10 minutes, stirring occasionally. Add in the remaining tablespoon of shortening and stir until it is fully incorporated.

5. Remove the caramel sauce from the heat and let it cool to room temperature before transferring it to a jar. Cover and refrigerate for up to 2 months. If the sauce solidifies it can be softened in the microwave.

TO SUBSTITUTE

Corn syrup (not high-fructose corn syrup) can be substituted for brown rice syrup.

Chocolate Syrup

You will want to use this rich chocolate syrup to top everything from frozen dessert sundaes to chocolate cake. Add it to non-dairy milk for a special breakfast (see page 33). This recipe makes dark chocolate syrup; use up to 2 tablespoons more sugar for a sweeter version.

½ cup plus 1 tablespoon (135 ml) Hemp Milk (page 31) or non-dairy milk of choice

2 tablespoons organic cane sugar

2 tablespoons brown rice syrup

½ teaspoon Vanilla Extract (page 288)

¼ cup (26 g) natural unsweetened cocoa powder

1 tablespoon chocolate chips

1 tablespoon shortening (see page 7)

1. Combine the milk, sugar, brown rice syrup, and vanilla in a medium saucepan. Heat over medium-low heat, until the sugars are melted.

2. Whisk in the cocoa and bring to a boil over medium heat. Boil until the mixture is smooth and slightly thickened, about 5 minutes.

3. Remove the pan from the heat and whisk in the chocolate chips and shortening until all of the ingredients are fully incorporated.

4. Let the chocolate syrup cool to room temperature before transferring it to a jar. Cover and refrigerate for up to 2 months.

TO SUBSTITUTE

Corn syrup (not high-fructose corn syrup) can be substituted for brown rice syrup.

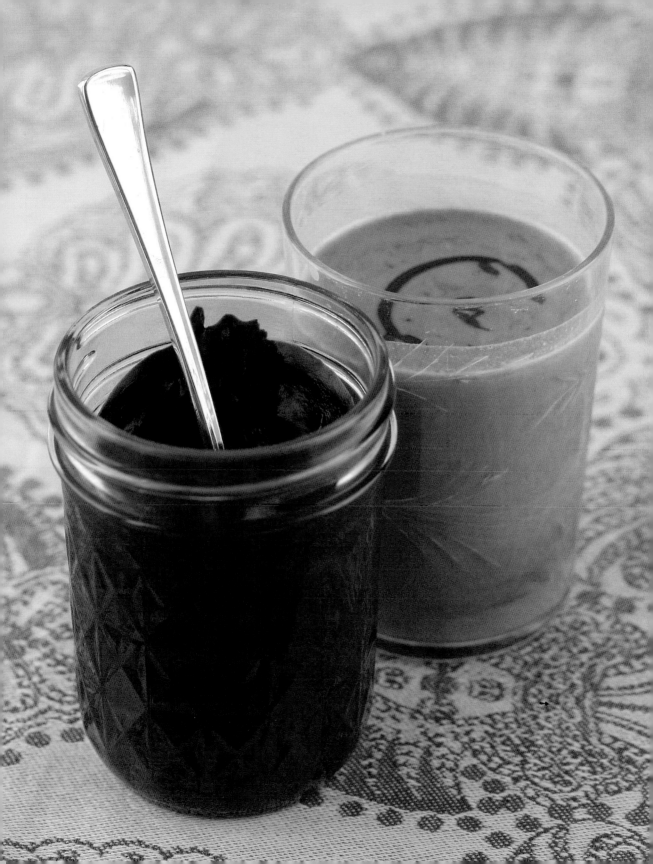

Vanilla Frosting

Whether you need just a little to make Chocolate Sandwich Cookies (page 241), or to decorate Brownie Bites (page 255), this frosting will cover them all. Always choose a firm shortening to make frosting (see page 7). If you plan to add Natural Food Coloring to vary the color and flavor, refer to page 295 before making the frosting.

3 cups (432 g) Powdered Sugar (page 286)

¼ teaspoon salt

1 tablespoon Vanilla Extract (page 288)

12 tablespoons shortening, softened (see page 7)

2 to 4 tablespoons water, as needed

1. Whisk together the powdered sugar and salt in a large mixing bowl to eliminate lumps. Add the vanilla and shortening and combine them using a mixer on medium-low speed until creamy, about 5 minutes. Scrape down the sides of the bowl as needed.

2. Add 2 tablespoons of water and mix on medium-low speed for 2 to 3 minutes, until the frosting is smooth. Add up to 2 more tablespoons of water as needed, ½ tablespoon at a time, until the desired consistency is reached.

3. Refrigerate for up to 1 month in an airtight container. If the frosting hardens in the refrigerator, let it sit at room temperature for up to 2 hours before using it; mix it together well to soften it.

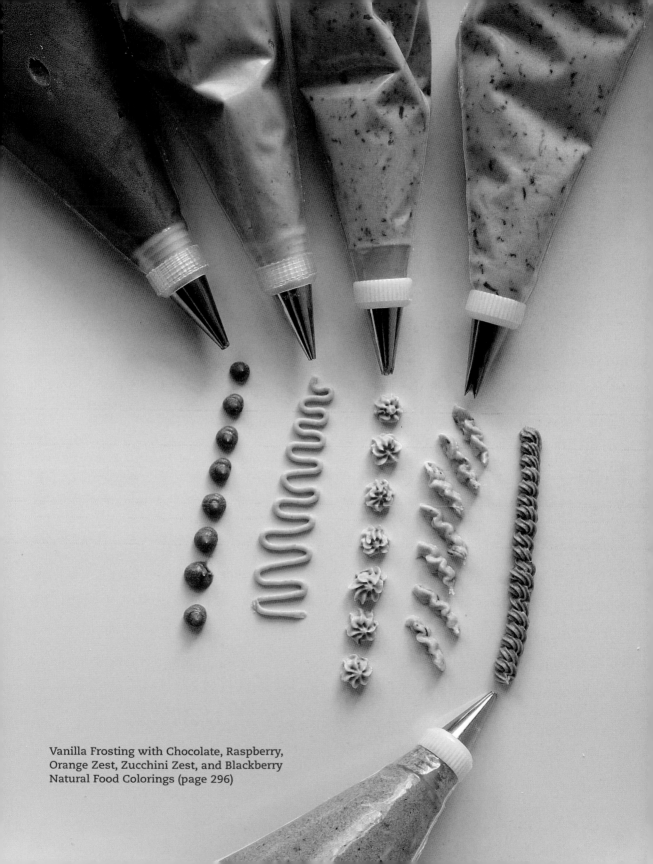

Vanilla Frosting with Chocolate, Raspberry,
Orange Zest, Zucchini Zest, and Blackberry
Natural Food Colorings (page 296)

Natural Food Colorings

I often wonder how we got comfortable consuming ingredients with names such as "yellow #5," or "blue #1," yet they appear in so many processed foods. Your doctor may advise you to avoid them or you may decide that your family is just better off without them. You always have the option to simply do without the color, but if you are inclined to make a cupcake look a little bit prettier, here's how you can do it with natural ingredients. The proportions listed here are to be used with the Vanilla Frosting recipe (page 294), which yields 2 cups (530 g) of frosting.

The colors achieved from these methods will be lighter than traditional food coloring. Also, keep in mind that the taste of the food you choose to make food coloring from will come across in the taste of the frosting—I consider that a benefit!

Berries

Berries are my favorite option for adding color to frosting; in addition to being able to achieve a medium-depth color, berries add nice flavor to frosting. One cup (150 g) of berries will provide between ¼ cup and ½ cup (60 ml and 120 ml) of food coloring. Food coloring made from berries should be refrigerated and used within 2 days. I do not recommend using bottled or canned juice to create color in frosting; the frosting will be too watery.

Pink: Raspberries or cranberries
Purple: Blackberries or very ripe blueberries

1. Wash and dry the berries. Puree them in a food processor and strain the puree through a fine mesh strainer to remove the pulp and seeds from the juice. The fruit coloring will be thick. (Save the pulp from the raspberries or blackberries to use as jam, if desired.)

2. To make frosting, add up to 4 tablespoons of fruit coloring (instead of 2 to 4 tablespoons of water) in step 2 on page 294. The amount of fruit coloring added will determine the depth of color in the frosting. Add the fruit coloring first, before adding any water to the frosting; it may not be needed.

Zest

Any citrus fruit with a skin can provide coloring. Vegetables with soft skins can also provide color; while technically this is not zest, the same technique is used to finely grate the skin. There will be small flecks of color in the frosting. Use zest on the same day as you prepare it.

Yellow: Orange zest (the zest from a lemon will be too light in color). One orange yields about 1 tablespoon of zest. (Squeeze the juice from the oranges to make a homemade glass of juice, if desired.)

Light Green: Lime zest. One lime yields about 1 teaspoon of zest.

Dark Green: Skin of a zucchini. One medium zucchini yields about 2 tablespoons of zest.

1. Wash the skins of the fruits or vegetables and dry them thoroughly. Use a microplane grater to finely grate the skin, being careful to zest only the top layer of the fruit or vegetable.
2. To make frosting, add up to 4 tablespoons of zest (in addition to the 2 to 4 tablespoons of water) in step 2 on page 294. The amount of zest added will determine the depth of the color in the frosting.

Chocolate

Because chocolate is fat, you must adjust the amount of shortening used in your frosting.

Brown or tan: Chocolate syrup

1. Reduce the amount of shortening in step 1 of the frosting recipe on page 294 to 8 tablespoons. Add 3 to 4 tablespoons of Chocolate Syrup (page 292).
2. Add 1 to 2 tablespoons of water (in addition to the 2 to 4 tablespoons of water in step 2 on page 294), as needed to achieve the desired consistency.

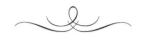

FLOUR WEIGHTS

Flour weights vary dramatically from brand to brand. Following are reference weights, by approximate volume.

FLOUR/STARCH	WEIGHT IN GRAMS			
	¼ CUP	½ CUP	¾ CUP	1 CUP
Amaranth	30	60	90	120
Brown rice	32	64	96	128
Buckwheat	40	80	120	160
Corn flour	29	58	87	116
Fava bean	33	66	99	132
Garbanzo bean	30	60	90	120
Masa harina	29	58	87	116
Millet	30	60	90	120
Oat	28	56	84	112
Potato flour	45	90	135	180
Quinoa	28	56	84	112
Sorghum	32	64	96	128
Sweet rice	30	60	90	120
White rice	32	64	96	128
Arrowroot starch	32	64	96	128
Corn starch	32	64	96	128
Potato starch	40	80	120	160
Tapioca starch	32	64	96	128

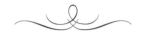

RESOURCES

NONPROFIT ORGANIZATIONS

These organizations provide education, support, and resources for individuals and families managing food allergies:

American Partnership for Eosinophilic Disorders (APFED)
apfed.org

The Asthma and Allergy Foundation of America (AAFA) and Kids with Food Allergies (KFA), a division of AAFA
aafa.org
kidswithfoodallergies.org

Food Allergy Research and Education (FARE)
foodallergy.org

TOOLS AND WEBSITES

Allergy Eats—An online and mobile guide to allergy-friendly restaurants.
allergyeats.com

Allergy Home—An online resource for awareness.
allergyhome.org

Asthma Allergies Children—A parent's web guide.
asthmaallergieschildren.com

SOURCES FOR INGREDIENTS

Amazon.com (various ingredients)
amazon.com

Authentic Foods (flours, starches, gums)
authenticfoods.com

Bob's Red Mill (flours, starches, and whole grains; may not be suitable for those with allergies to soy and tree nuts)
bobsredmill.com/Gluten-Free

Divvies Bakery (chocolate; may not be suitable for those with allergies to soy)
divvies.com

Earth Balance (shortening and spreads)
earthbalancenatural.com

Enjoy Life (chocolate)
enjoylifefoods.com

King Arthur Flour (flours, starches, gums)
kingarthurflour.com/glutenfree

Living Harvest (hemp milk and hemp products)
livingharvest.com

Nu Life Market (sorghum flour)
nulifemarket.com

Nutiva (coconut oil, hemp seeds, chia seeds)
nutiva.com

So Delicious Dairy Free (coconut milk and coconut milk products)
sodeliciousdairyfree.com/products

Spectrum Organics (coconut oil, palm fruit oil, other oils, flax seeds)
spectrumorganics.com/index.php

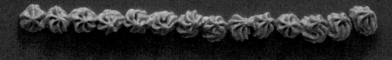

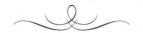

ACKNOWLEDGMENTS

Every book is a work of art that can only come together with the hard work, dedication, and support of a team. My agent, Steve Troha, championed the book. Matthew Lore and Cara Bedick agreed to take the project on at The Experiment. Molly Cavanaugh, my uber-talented editor, helped to bring my vision to life. Erica Ferguson made sure I had all my commas in the right place and Joanna Williams designed a mouthwatering cover. Pauline Neuwirth and her associates transformed my photos and words into a creative masterpiece. Karen Giangreco created the e-book in various digital formats. Dan O'Connor, Anne Rumberger, Sarah Schneider, and the team at Workman Publishing all helped to make the book a success. Thank you all.

Thank you to the friends and family who supported this effort, tried (and tried again) recipes until they were perfect, and put up with my obsessive behavior and gluten-free flour flying around the kitchen. Special thanks to my husband, Harry, who happily taste-tested crackers for ten days in a row and didn't complain when he couldn't find the top of the dining room table. Thank you to Kevin and Patrick for your encouragement and inspiration. I love you all.

As I have pursued my work to help families with multiple food allergies, I have found a truly supportive and welcoming community that I am privileged to be a part of. This community, made up of food-allergy parents, bloggers, authors, entrepreneurs, medical professionals, and advocates inspires me every day. Special thanks to those who give freely of their time and resources to help advance awareness, drive legislation, and educate those around them about food allergies, eosinophilic gastrointestinal disorders, and celiac disease.

Last, I must thank the readers of my website, *Learning to Eat Allergy-Free*, and my first book, *Learning to Bake Allergen-Free*, as well as those of you reading this book. You are the reason I continue to develop recipes, share my knowledge, and write books. You make it all worthwhile.

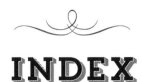

INDEX

Note: Page references in **bold italics** indicate recipe photographs.

proofing dough, 49
Pudding, Chocolate, 278, **279**

Q

quick-rising yeast, 49
Quinoa Bowl, 192, **193**
quinoa flour, 299

R

Raisin Chocolate Granola Bars, **138**, 139
Ranch Dressing, Dairy-Free, **108**, 109
Raspberry Fruit Roll-Ups, **276**, 277
Raspberry Maple Syrup, **119**, 121
Raspberry Vinaigrette, 102
rice flours, 19, 299
Rice Milk, 32
rice milk, powdered, 10
rolling pins, 219
Rolls, Dinner, 56, **57**

S

salads
    Asian-Inspired Coleslaw, **150**, 151
    Caesar Salad, **154**, 155
    Croutons for, 64, **65**
    Polenta Croutons for, **66**, 67
    Potato Salad, 148, **149**
Salsa, **195**, 214, **215**
salt, 10
Sandwich Bread, **50**, 51
Sandwich Cookies, Chocolate, **240**, 241–42
Sandwiches, Non-Dairy Ice Cream, **264**, 265–66
sauces
    Barbecue Sauce, 110, **111**
    Caramel Sauce, **290**, 291
    Cauliflower Cream and Creamed Vegetables, **146**, 147
    Cheesy Sauce, **175**, 176
    Honey Mustard Sauce, **112**, 113, **190**, **207**

Marinara Sauce, 178, **179**
    Pesto, **57**, **171**, 177
    Salsa, **195**, 214, **215**
Scones, Apple Oatmeal, 124, **125**
seed grinders, 43
seeds
    as egg substitutes, 41
    See also specific seeds
Shepherd's Pie, 188, **189**
shortenings, 7
sides
    Asian-Inspired Coleslaw, **150**, 151
    Baked Beans, 152, **153**
    Caesar Salad, **154**, 155
    Cauliflower Cream and Creamed Vegetables, **146**, 147
    French Fries, **158**, 159
    Fried Batter Mix and Onion Rings, **162**, 163–64
    Fried Polenta Sticks, 160, **161**
    Potato Puffs, 156, **157**
    Potato Salad, 148, **149**
    silicone molds, 37
    Simple Vinaigrette, 102, **103**
snacks
    Buckwheat Maple Crackers, 228, **229**
    Buttery Crackers, 224, **225**
    Dill Pickles, **208**, 209
    Flax Crackers, **83**, **222**, 223
    Hummus, **69**, **212**, 213, **230**
    Pita Chips, **230,** 231
    Potato Chips, 210, **211**
    Salsa, **195**, 214, **215**
    Soft-Baked Pretzel Bites, 206, **207**
    Spicy Hemp Crackers, **226**, 227
Snickerdoodles, **244**, 245
Soft-Baked Pretzel Bites, 206, **207**
sorghum flour, 19, 23, 299
Soup, Potato Leek, **198**, 199

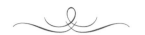

ABOUT THE AUTHOR

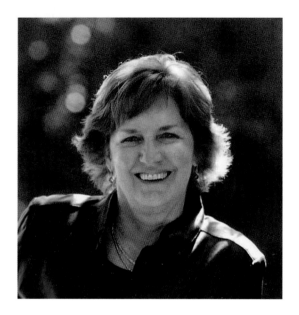

Colette Martin is a food-allergy advocate, an expert on how to bake allergen-free, and the author of the critically acclaimed *Learning to Bake Allergen-Free: A Crash Course for Busy Parents on Baking without Wheat, Gluten, Dairy, Eggs, Soy or Nuts.* When her son was diagnosed with multiple food allergies, she had to reinvent how her family ate. Having first learned to bake in her grandmother's kitchen with wheat, butter, milk, and eggs,

Colette understands firsthand what it means to transform her kitchen to accommodate multiple food allergies. She is a member of the Kids with Food Allergies advisory board.

You can find her website, *Learning to Eat Allergy-Free*, at www.learningtoeatallergyfree. com, follow her on Twitter @colettefmartin, like her on facebook.com/allergenfreebaker, or e-mail her at multifoodallergies@gmail.com.